Ask Your Body

*Relieve Your Food Allergies Instantly
and Naturally with Muscle Testing*

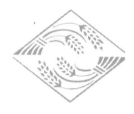

Elizabeth F. Spicer Ph.D.

MEDICINE BEAR PUBLISHING
BLUE HILL, MAINE

Ask Your Body: Relieve Your Food Allergies
Instantly and Naturally with Muscle Testing
by
Elizabeth F. Spicer Ph.D.

Published in 1998

Photographs by: Holly English-Payne
Cover Art by: Elizabeth F. Spicer

Published by:

Medicine Bear Publishing
P.O. Bx 1075
Blue Hill, ME 0461

ISBN# 1-891850-09-1
Library of Congress CCN# 98-06753

A Preliminary Note to the Reader

In a nutshell, this book will teach you how to communicate with your body. It will give you a valuable tool, a simple, safe method for testing any food, medicine or substance, before eating it, taking it, or washing with it, to see if it will weaken you. Hives, indigestion, migraines, hyperactivity, exhaustion after meals and long term illnesses such as arthritis, are often related to food sensitivities that no one would ever suspect. Sensitivities to medication can produce dangerous side effects. With the tool of muscle testing, you can determine these sensitivities easily and accurately.

Muscle testing provided me with a totally reliable tool for keeping myself hives-free during the years I was highly allergic, and it gave me a safe and pain-free way of learning when my allergies were subsiding. It allowed me to maximize my diet at all times, and to live, unmedicated, without horrible ugly burning red blotches on my face and hands. I have spent the last four years studying and refining the technique, to understand it fully, to troubleshoot it and to be certain one could control for any possible inaccuracies. I am thrilled and impressed with its power and grateful for the control it can give.

For children, especially, whose allergies cause not only physical pain, but also emotional stigma and a life touched by fear, and for their long-suffering parents, this book puts you and your child back in control. Imagine a testing method that is easy, painless, even fun — a game you play together. Imagine being able to find out exactly what is and is not safe, anytime, anywhere you need to know. Imagine being able to take your child off medication, because you finally know exactly what to avoid and what to replace it with. Muscle testing can instantly turn your situation around, allowing you all to live more normally, fear-free. Your child can once again see the world as a friendly and negotiable place.

If you are someone who truly is attracted to the idea of learning a simple but powerful technique, and taking complete control and responsibility for the knowledge you gain in the process — then read on and learn!

Table of Contents

Help yourself and your family

How muscle testing saved my skin and my sanity; Fran's stomach attacks, Michael's migraines; Mom's Stories—Arthritis and Overdose; The flatulent six year old; The teenager who listened to her body—not her mother; Teen alcoholism — could addiction be a form of allergy?; Camp food; Holistic health in reverse

I am not allergic—Why would I want to know about muscle testing?

Will I react to the medicine?; Adoptive parents; Is the green food in the fridge safe?; Restaurant dining—for better or worse; Is overweight an allergic reaction?; Camping out—eating off the land; Vitamin dosages; Irritable bowel and hiatus hernia; Testing newborns; Nutritionists; Geriatric Physicians; Personal trainers; Psychotherapists

Is this scientific?

The search for decaf; The Scientific Method and the ricotta cheese mystery; Times I doubted it; Conclusion

Why doesn't the world already know about this?

Western culture and medicine—attitudes and paradigm shifts; Our feelings about our bodies and our doctors; It is not good business for anyone; Professionals who do use muscle testing; "Undependable"—inaccuracies and incomplete information

Chapter 5
Learning the method and its variations
The Basic (Arm) method; Troubleshooting (Bouncing arms, positions and the sex factor, accidental short circuiting, subject becomes too "strong"); Alternate testing methods for special situations (discreet methods, surrogate testing, self-testing); What else do I need to know?

Chapter 6

How does it work?
Energy fields; Eastern medicine and body circuitry; Why?—is another question

Chapter 7

What do the results mean?
Individual answers; Stomach intolerance; Allergic types of response; Long term problems; Momentary weakness; The role of quantity; Location and amount

Chapter 8

What should I test?
Subgroups and brands; Hidden foods, Portions; Being ready for change, Medications and supplements; One person's cure is another one's poison; Nonfoods (latex, soaps, lotions, perfumes)

Chapter 9

Living happily with the results
Coping with limitations and realizing possibilities; Making lists; Surviving and enjoying restaurants; Holiday gift packs; Children's happiness

Medical Disclaimer

This book will teach you to use a tool, which will empower you to make decisions about what you or others might eat or use. Any decisions you make based on the use of this tool are your own decisions. You are in control, and with control comes responsibility. Therefore, you are responsible for any decisions or actions taken as a result of your own testing, as well as any consequences of them.

No medical advice is being given in this book. If you or others have any medical problem involving allergies or other food intolerance, which requires medical attention, consult with your doctor before making any changes in diet or medication.

Preface

You have just begun a journey that could dramatically change your life, and perhaps that of one you hold dear! This succinct, beautifully written volume will teach you everything you need to know to determine whether a given substance should be eaten...or whether it could cause harmful effects.

If your needs are urgent, you could get the "how to" manual by turning directly to Chapter 5. If you have a little more time, and are curious about the origins of muscle testing, how Dr. Spicer, a college mathematics professor came to learn about it, and whom she encountered along the way, I suggest that you continue from here. Dr. Spicer has the curiosity of a scientist, the logic of a mathematician, and the writing gift of a mystery story author.

Ask Your Body teaches us about muscle testing and kinesiology, the how's, the why's, the what's, the when's and the wherefore's. Dr Spicer does not stop there. She explains why it has not been accepted before and heads off the skeptic and quackbuster before they can affect anyone with a sincere quest for Truth. If this were not enough, our author then proceeds to teach a simple form of desensitization and even gives a treatment for those who discover a little late that they have inadvertently ingested a deleterious substance.

I must admit that I have been using a crude form of muscle testing in my practice for several years. Once I even used it on a patient that I had admitted to a local teaching hospital. A colleague, who has a specialty practice in New York City, asked me to hospitalize a Long Island teenager for whom he was caring. She had had such abdominal pains at times, that he was pushed to using pain killer injections. While making rounds one night, (I doubt that I would have had the courage during the day), I decided to try muscle testing for various substances. Lo and behold, I found one drug that was quite benign, and which proved to be very effective when taken orally! Consequently, I've been a believer for some time...but this book has enhanced my comfort level, accuracy, and ability to explain the use of muscle testing to my patients and their parents, who laugh and agree that it's weird...but who have the trust, faith and love to want to help themselves and their families.

I highly recommend that every openminded man, woman and child become familiar with the material in this book. I trust that those parents and physicians who are at the cutting edge of 21st century medicine, will benefit from Elizabeth Spicer's endeavor to share her life enhancing discoveries.

— Diane Acker M.D., F.A.A.P.

Chapter I

Help yourself and your family

This book contains a gift. For those people who need it urgently, it can feel more like a miracle. For others it may be simply a useful tool for getting information. As for me, it was a turning point in my life, that saved me from a desperation that would have sent me over the edge.

The technique you will learn from this book rescued me from months of suffering from unknown food allergies, suddenly putting me back in control of my life and allowing me to go off heavy medication. It then helped my husband to tiptoe around a diet which has minimized his migraines, my mother to forestall developing arthritis and eliminate adverse reactions to medication, and my niece to end a long-standing series of stomach pain attacks. On the lighter side, it has also helped my sister to lose the ten pounds she never could get rid of before.

Outside my immediate family, it has turned around the life of a teenager who had accepted his stomach problems as a fact of life, a child who had always been "sickly", a college girl who refused to listen to her mother but was very willing to listen to her body, and a dropout who found her addiction to beer might really have been a type of food intolerance. It has even given some relief to a six year old who had been troubled by excessive flatulence.

Why are allergies and food sensitivities becoming so increasingly prevalent in the population today? How can we strengthen our bodies to become less allergic or sensitive? There are many theories and excellent books available that seek to answer these questions. Their foundations range from traditional medicine, to holistic, alternative, or complimentary therapies. This book will not attempt to enter these discussions, or pretend to tell you, the reader, what to do or not to do in your life. What you will gain from this book is the tool, the technique you can use to come to your own decisions. And you will gain the benefit of my years of experience, that have opened my eyes to understandings and possibilities for the use of this tool that would not occur to the more casual user.

In this chapter, you will see how muscle testing has helped people in a variety of circumstances. Perhaps you will see yourself or someone in your family in one of these situations.

How Muscle Testing saved my skin and my sanity:

One Monday morning in March 1994, I awoke with a a painful burning on my face and hands, went to the mirror and gasped at the swollen-nosed, red blotchy person looking back at me. I then noticed that my hands and arms were covered with what looked like a bad case of eczema. It was the beginning of what would be a five month nightmare. I had suddenly become allergic to most of the normal foods people eat.

Initially, I was not aware that I had allergies. It took a while to determine that food was even the problem, because I was reactive to so many different foods that cutting out some suspicious ones did not help. Nevertheless, the day I had tomato soup for lunch, and fifteen minutes later my hands exploded hot and red, I knew in my heart that foods were the cause.

The dermatologist winced when he saw my distorted face and bumpy hands and arms. He told me, not surprisingly, that I was having a severe allergic response. But strangely, when I went to allergists, the skin tests were repeatedly negative, even for foods that were definitely causing the hives, and negative again for all other foods I suspected. No allergies. Call it by another name, no one could deny the swollen red burning blotches. I was subsequently tested for all sorts of medical problems, but came out with a clean slate. All we could do was treat the symptoms.

For weeks I was on and off antihistamines at high dosages. I even took steroids to try and control the pain, burning, and itching. At best they were only partly helpful. I tried to conduct my normal life, both for myself and my five year old, but in a constant state of severe physical discomfort, my mood could be best described as rotten. I felt ugly and conspicuous, as I noticed people do a little double take when they saw my distorted red face and arms. My students were polite, but I could see they were somewhat taken aback by my appearance. It was unlike me to take heavy medication, but there seemed to be no other choice. The burning hives would move from place to place on my body, but never completely go away. Some nights my hands throbbed and burned so badly that I could only sleep with wet towels wrapped around them. Would I ever look and feel normal again? Why wouldn't it just finish up and go away? How long could this last? And what was wrong with me anyway? I was starting to lose my emotional grip.

In desperation, I tried cutting my diet down to five innocuous foods. Finally, I began to see a change, my skin started to come back, and I began gradually to feel like a human being again. Only then was I able to go off the medications. My skin returned to an almost normal state. At least this proved it was a food allergy after all. But how long could I live on five foods? Would I ever be able to go to a restaurant again? If only I had some way of knowing what I was allergic to!

After complete medical testing I had been told my only option was to go on antihistamines for a year. I knew that would not work for me. At that point I gave up on a medical solution. I would have to handle it with diet. There was not much left I dared eat, but at least I had stopped assaulting my body with the medication, and I was comfortable. Having given up on anyone else to help me, at least I was in partial control. The biggest problem was that I had no idea what was safe to eat, and no way to find out except by trial and too often painful error. I will never forget the feeling I had the day I took my daughter into Manhattan, to Radio City Music Hall, to see the Lion King. Feeling as if I were in a strange nightmarish reality, we went from one restaurant to another looking for someplace to eat lunch. I was then confronted with the fact that I could not eat one entree on any of the menus —anywhere!

In July, I received what I now view as a miracle. My sister, Barbara, recalled something we had first encountered in the late Seventies, then called "Muscle Response Testing." A fellow named Don had been using it to determine what kinds of vitamins and supplements people needed to strengthen their bodies against all kinds of ills. He was locally well known and had supposedly helped many people with dramatic results. More recently, a chiropractor had used it on me, in Barbara's presence, to try to determine what parts of my body were weak and perhaps causing the hives. We wondered if we could use it to test for weakness to foods. The method seemed like hocus-pocus, but desperate situations lead to desperate solutions, and so we tried it on me. Thank heavens, Barbara was naturally adept at testing. For the first time, I tested weak to tomatoes and strong to lettuce, confirming the truth.

And what was this miracle of muscle testing? A firm downward push on my outstretched arm, while I held a food in front of my stomach* with the other hand. When I held the tomato, it was as if there were no muscle to resist a push. My arm went right down with barely any pressure on it. When I held the lettuce and she tried the same push, I suddenly had plenty of strength to keep my arm outstretched and resist the pressure downward.

Amazed and thrilled, we tried the test on every food we knew

---

*I have always told people to put their hand on their *stomach, gut,* or *tummy.* and everyone had a good "gut" feeling for where that was. However, doctors have corrected me, explaining that the stomach is actually over to the left side. Therefore, the more medically accurate term might be "upper abdomen." It is the area one gets "stomach aches." that is at or just below the bellybutton. Let us agree that the word for this spot will be "stomach" in all future descriptions in this book, and I beg pardon from the doctors for using the term very loosely.

about, and got accurate results. Had we stumbled on a way of directly asking my body what would be okay or problematic, without my having to eat anything first and suffer? I jumped around the room screaming crazily. Could this be true? The panic I had felt for months began to subside. Food would no longer be a horror, just a big, but controllable inconvenience. We wondered, how could such an incredibly easy, free gift from Nature be so unknown and unavailable?

I began to go back to restaurants. This was a major healing process for me. My sister became my indispensable eating companion. We tested whole plates of food. I could not have cared less about how it looked to others. My husband started to learn how to test me. This took a bit of time, but eventually he got the technique.

One day the impossible happened - I tested strong for a plate of Shrimp Scampi. My original hives attack had followed a very large shrimp cocktail, and I had avoided shrimp for months. Could I trust it? I took a deep breath, and a small bite. An hour later I was still fine. That evening I found out I could eat such exotic things as garlic crabs and lobster. Ecstatic, I added seafood to my increasing repertoire. How could I have ever known about these possibilities any other way?

I became passionate about spreading the word to others who might also be suffering. When we arose to test plates of food, and fellow diners would chuckle or stare, I would take the opportunity to explain, or offer to teach them the method to use on anyone they knew who needed help. I was surprised to find out how many people had some degree of food sensitivity.

Meanwhile, acquaintances thought I had suddenly "gotten better." I certainly looked better, and I appeared to be eating more normally. But my close friends knew it was really my own strange miracle, this muscle testing. Some dismissed me as nuts, but those with their own allergies were more open-minded and were also amazed and impressed. More than one person implied politely that it may be all in my mind, that I became reactive to foods when I was made nervous by a weak muscle test or suspicious of a food. To those people I told this little story, which I now call *"Shelley Creamcheese."*

I was having lunch with my friend Shelley who was visiting me, Because of the food reactions, I apologetically suggested we stay at the house and just have something innocuous like a bagel and cream cheese. As I was finishing, perhaps twenty minutes into lunch, I started brushing aside what felt like a hair against my nose. But the hair would not go away, because it was not there. With a sinking feeling, I recognized it as the first sign of the hives, which came back and plagued me for three days thereafter. Originally, I was not nervous whatsoever about that cream cheese, and I really could not believe it was the culprit either, until the next day when we were testing everything I had eaten the day before, and the muscle test made it crystal clear. I would never have suspected cream cheese. Why was it a problem when milk was not a problem?

There were many strange, inexplicable facts that eventually emerged, things I will never understand, but accepted because they "just were." Why was I only able to eat green apples and not red ones? Why was a certain ginger ale strong and another weak? Why could I eat only the black nubby avocados and not the shiny green ones? Why were onions a problem and leeks okay? Why I could eat only a certain brand of black forest ham, and no other brand I tested? Why only white fish and not dark or pink ones? Why in the world was one brand of cheese not a problem, when every other hard cheese was? And how in the world could I ever have gotten this information from any doctor, even if skin testing *had* worked for me? What we had here was an amazingly powerful and useful tool, a tool to change lives. I was thrilled with the discovery.

In an effort to figure out what was wrong with me, I tried collecting as much information as I could in a very long list of good and bad foods, hoping that by presenting it to an allergist we could ferret out the real nature of the physical problem. A doctor friend gave me the name of a top notch person, who had "written the book" on the subject and to whom he sent all his unusual cases. At my appointment, he insisted on doing another series of skin tests of a slightly different nature. I went along with it, just to prove to him that those tests really were not working for me. And they were not. Even so, after that, he seemed to have little interest in my lists, and told me I should come back for more skin testing! I tried to explain that I really did not need a way of determining the foods I was allergic to, thanks to the kinesiology (the name chiropractors use for it); but it became obvious that he held no stock in my testing or my information. As you might suspect, I did not make the appointment for more skin testing. It was at this point that I came to my eventual philosophy on food sensitivities, "Forget about why, and just feel better!" I thanked heaven twice, because I now my own answers.

The fact is, I used muscle testing intensively for over two years, testing perhaps five to ten items on any given day, and I never got a false result. As my own allergies began to subside (a subject discussed more in *Chapter Twelve*), the muscle tests became harder to read, which corresponded with the fact that my reactions to offending foods were becoming less intense. Once muscle testing entered my life, the only times I ever again had to endure those awful hives were when I made a mistake, and neglected to test something by assuming it was safe. And even then, I was always able to find out what had caused the problem by testing everything I had eaten the day before.

As of the writing of this book, my own food sensitivities have dwindled down to just a few. I still test at restaurants, just to be sure, and also to locate hidden ingredients. I am often surprised to find something in the recipe I did not suspect. Even if I eventually become totally non-allergic, muscle testing will always be an active part of my life.

Fran's Stomach Attacks:

It was the evening I discovered I could eat shrimp scampi—a banner day in my life. Joining us at the restaurant that night were Barbara's son Eric, my nephew, and his wife Fran. Eric was 25 then, a great guy — sharp, macho, but sensitive. As he watched his mom test me, he began to chuckle. When he saw my thrill at being able to eat shrimp, he smiled and said, "Well, if you believe in that sort of thing." I was jolted into action. "This is no belief system!," I roared, "This is truth!"

I then told him my entire story, quickly but with great intensity. Fortunately, he had enough respect for me to listen; he knows me as the professor with the Ph.D., down to earth and logical. Also, since I was not his mother, he was likely more willing to accept what I was saying. After a while, he said, "You know, Franny has been having some stomach problems..." It seemed she had been having severe stomach cramps every night for some months, and that she was in such pain, she had made an appointment to have a GI series.

Well, as they say, the rest is history. Together Barbara and I convinced the group to spend Saturday evening at the supermarket. We tested Fran for just about anything we could think of, and especially for the foods she had always suspected. We found she was very weak for all dairy and red meats, as well as tomato sauce. So much for the pizza she ate so frequently, and the steaks she had never been partial to, but had started eating since she married Eric, a steak lover. We also determined which brands of margarine and lactose-free milk were safe for her to have. Half-believing, she stopped drinking milk, and stayed away from all the other problem foods we had discovered, although she did have some cheese. That night, for the first time in months, she only had a mild case of stomach pain. Having more faith in the testing procedure, she then strictly cut out all offending foods and anything made with them. That was the end of her problem. And a month or so later, rather than being in the midst of extensive medical testing, she became happily and healthily pregnant. Often, when I look at Adam, my grand-nephew, now three years old, I do thank God for muscle testing even more than before.

Just a postscript on Fran. She continued to stay mostly off problem foods for some months and found that her sensitivities decreased over time. Pregnancy also reduced her allergies. Now she has incorporated most of the changes easily into her life style, and understands that if she binges too much she will have to deal with the consequences. Most importantly, she is in control.

Michael's Migraines:

My husband, Michael, although he accepted the concept of muscle testing, did not become totally comfortable with it right away. Living with me, he was faced daily with its reliability for my situation, but in retrospect, it took a while for him to fully " know" that the technique was easy and reliable in general. It also took quite some time before he took over as my major tester. I think he was not anxious to become my tester at first because he did not want to be responsible for the consequences in case something went wrong. But he was game to try, and we kept attempting to do the testing on foods I already knew about, just as practice. After some weeks, he gained accuracy and confidence, and it became clear his readings could be trusted. It was then that I became really free. Now we could go out with anyone, not just my sister and brother-in-law, and I could have some dinner choices at any restaurant.

During those weeks, he became interested in knowing how he would test to some foods, and asked Barbara to try testing him. Michael has always had a fairly sensitive stomach, and migraines for many years, and we had always suspected foods might have been triggers for stomach distress or the headaches. Over years, we had noticed that the day after Thanksgiving, he had a migraine. Even the day after I had made something as healing as chicken soup, he had a migraine. I recall one day, years ago, we were saying, "Do you think it could be the chicken?" and then both of us, "Naaaah!"

In an attempt to find out exactly what foods might be better avoided, two years previously, Michael had gone to an allergist who did a very complex, and terribly expensive (approximately $1000) series of Rast allergy blood tests. His results indicated no significant response to any of the foods or substances included in the test, and so we had no useable information from that source. Would muscle testing give any results?

What we got were dramatic results. It turned out that when he held chocolate, his other arm had no muscle strength at all. He had the same weakness with peanuts and American cheese. All these are commonly known as migraine producing, but his allergy test did not find them. Most interestingly, when he held chicken or turkey of any kind, uncooked, cooked, white, dark, his arm sunk down immediately. At the suggestion of a friend, we tried organic chicken, thinking the problem might have been the chemicals introduced by processing. Still weak. So much for the post Thanksgiving migraines.

On the other hand, he tested perfectly strong for regular coffee, and soda, although decaf and diet soda with chemical sweeteners were no good. Later on we learned that certain artificial sweeteners are often a trigger for migraines, and that some sufferers get relief by having caffeine. So perhaps we would have eventually found out about those drinks without muscle testing. But by testing we knew exactly what to do for him even before we knew why. It takes a leap of faith in our reason-oriented society to accept that we can get and use information without knowing the reason it works, but that is the leap of faith both my husband and I eventually made. At that point in time he became a total convert to muscle testing as a way of life. As time went on, he discovered that many foods he was never particularly drawn toward (i.e. chicken) were really not good for him. Also some foods he craved in an almost addictive way (such as chocolate). Now when we went to restaurants it was a double process. I would test him for anything on his plate and he would then test me. People watching us began to think we were from some kind of religious cult.

I would love to say that his migraines disappeared forever at that point, but that is just not true. His situation was not as black and white as mine. Probably migraine is a complex mechanism that can be triggered by food, but that does not mean that eliminating the food triggers will wipe out the whole problem. What I can honestly say is that he has fewer headaches and they do not seem to be as devastating as they used to be. Certainly, we are eliminating the cause of many potential problems for him.

Mom's Stories - Arthritis and Overdose:

My mother had been with us all in 1978 when we first witnessed Don's muscle testing, and she, like we, had accepted the possibility that it might actually be doing something. But she was never completely convinced. Recently, my sister had been after her for some time to stop eating the food group called "nightshades," which contained some of her favorite foods such as potato, tomato, green pepper and eggplant. According to the holistic literature, the night-shade group is a cause of arthritis; and my mother has had, off and on during periods of time, somewhat disabling arthritis since she was in her fifties. During the summer of 1994, while all this was happening to me, she was having rather painful arthritis in her hand and she finally submitted to testing. Immediately we found out she should not be having tomatoes or green peppers. She really did not want to know about this, since these vegetables had been a mainstay for her, and she had been losing weight by eating what she felt was a very "healthful" diet of pasta, with her own home-made tomato-vegetable mixture on it. By her own admission, she craved tomatoes, and really did not want to have to cut them out of her diet. She would not accept this truth until we showed her repeatedly that while she was strong for a multitude of other foods, including eggplant, tomatoes were definitely no good.

A notable point came through at that time. Muscle testing could be used to indicate foods that bring on no momentary symptoms, but are the cause of a chronic type of problem, like arthritis. My mother never had a sudden attack of any kind after eating tomatoes. It must have been a gradual weakening process that was being indicated. Again, if we were looking for a black and white verification of the truth in muscle test results, it would not be available here. But after witnessing my accuracy and success, and her own extremely weak response to the push on her arm (her whole body would lean to a side and almost topple when the arm was pushed), it became clear to us all that tomatoes were weakening her and she finally agreed to stop eating them.

That also meant stopping all tomato products, (ketchup, soup and pizza) but she did it, with very few exceptions. She also stopped eating green peppers. We noticed some weeks later, before she was aware of it, that she was starting to use her right hand more than she had been before. Very gradually that round of arthritis eased up. Would it have happened anyway? We cannot prove that going off tomatoes and peppers helped her then, but it certainly seemed that way.

She did insist that we retest her for tomatoes from time to time. She really missed them and kept wishfully thinking that if she stayed off them for some time maybe she could start eating them again. My sister and I doubted it, but we indulged her, and tested her every so often. One day I was testing her and she was suddenly strong for the can of tomato sauce that generally weakened her. Amazed, we repeated the test on other tomato products and found a consistently strong response. She was thrilled. "I knew it!," she announced triumphantly. Green peppers were still a no-no, but that did not matter. When she started to order the veal parmigiana again, my sister and I worried and tested her, but the test kept confirming that it was still good for her to eat. Since then, she has kept her tomato consumption moderate with no more binging for weeks straight eating ratatouille, and she has continued to test strong.

A second notable point emerged from this experience—Keep retesting for any changes that may have occurred. Since the test is so easy and fast, and can be done anytime you and a tester are together, retesting can be done as often as you would like to know an answer.

Now, years later, the arthritis has been off and on, but seems to be not as severe as it had been. We continue to test, and we get information that leads to a diet that she will follow willingly, if not happily. Interestingly, green peppers never strengthened up at all for her, so she uses red ones instead. Those are not considered nightshades, and she has always tested strong for them. Of the four nightshade vegetables, potatoes and eggplant never tested weak. Again here, we had gotten some of this information from my sister, and practitioners of alternative medicine do advise against eating those four vegetables if one is an arthritis sufferer. But by asking her own body for personal information, we were able to see which of the four were actually problematic for her, and which ones she could eat without concern. I am still impressed.

At the time I began writing this book, the above story was going to be the total "Mom's Story" section. However, something much more crucial, even life-threatening, took place since that time. It was a series of events that drove the point home powerfully that we all need muscle testing to be available in our lives, allergic or not.

Mom's Story 2:

It was the morning of New Year's Day, 1996. My family visited my sister's family to celebrate New Year's Eve quietly, and had slept over. We had spoken to my mother earlier in the evening from her condominium in Florida, and she told us that she felt fantastic and was about to go out dancing. We chuckled at the call. She had been taking a fair dose of prednisone for a few days, prescribed by a physician to relieve a case of hives she got after taking a certain pain killer for arthritis pain. I knew from my own experience with prednisone that it had made me quite cheerful and lively during the weeks I took it and I firmly believe it contributed to my sudden allergies after I stopped, but that is another story. So for a few days she had been calling very animatedly to tell me that she had taken some nice brisk walks and had cleaned up her apartment to perfection, and I recognized the "high" as she spoke uncharacteristically quickly in a non-stop rush of lively chatter.

At 8 AM, New Year's morning, we awoke to a phone call that jarred us out of slumber. It was my mother, in Florida, with panic in her voice, breathlessly telling us that an ambulance was about to take her away to the hospital, and that her heart was jumping around wildly with a runaway heartbeat rate. She had insisted on calling us even as they held her on a stretcher, and I was terrified at the tone in her voice. It had been three years since my father died, but my mother had seemed to be so strong and vital, especially for the previous few days. We all went into shock as we spent the next hour frantically on the phone trying to keep track of her location and her progress, so that we could have a hand in any decisions that were being made, so far away.

I had told her it had to be the Prednisone, which had made her too high, and now had taxed her body to this point. She thought so too, and that thought calmed her somewhat, as it implied that this was not an occurrence caused by her age or physical condition so much as a bad side effect of a medication. While the first two doctors refused to confirm that heart arrhythmia was a possible side effect of prednisone, a third finally was honest enough to agree. By then we had looked it up in the P.D.R. (physician's desk reference) anyway and found out ourselves.

Thank heavens the doctors in the hospital found something to give her that ended the attack. We all breathed a sigh of relief, in New York and Florida. She seemed all right, but they wanted her to stay in the hospital for observation. I knew immediately I had to fly down, not only to give her some outside-the-hospital control, but more importantly, to muscle test her for anything they wanted to medicate her with in the hospital. It had become painfully obvious to us, after several instances of bad reactions to medicines and now this reaction to prednisone, that my mother was very sensitive to medication and likely to have side effects. I was extremely grateful we had a tool like muscle testing on our side. While she waited the day for me to come down, she had to refuse prednisone several times, as nurses who had been given her a list of medications attempted to give her more.

When I got down the next day and tested her, the results were totally clear. Even a small bit of prednisone weakened her completely. I wished that I or someone had been there to test her, before she took it in the first place. I truly believe that if she had been tested daily for the few days she was taking it, a weak test would have shown up.

In the days that followed, we refused certain possible medications and accepted others, all on the basis of the testing. It had been an invaluable tool in keeping her body from danger, and as far as I was concerned, had completely proven itself to be crucial basic knowledge for everyone, allergic or not.

As a postscript to this story, the hives mentioned earlier developed into a painful and ugly blistering skin disease which occasionally afflicts older people, and while we fought the use of prednisone until she could stand the symptoms no longer, it was prednisone that eventually relieved her. In determining a safe dosage, we used muscle testing constantly to check as she very slowly worked her system up to the necessary level. (Her previous experience had been after starting at a high level with no buildup time.) She actually was able, under the controlled buildup using muscle testing, to safely accept higher levels of it than the ones that had previously sent her body over the edge. And we all had the peace of mind of knowing that each successive increment was still testing strong.

The flatulent six year old:

Let us switch from a very serious situation to an almost frivolous but still important effect of muscle testing. It involved my daughter's playmate Amy, whose mother had become increasingly upset as her little girl suffered from flatulence. OK, so it was only farting, but it had gotten to the point where her mom was torn between embarrassment and concern about her daughter's health. She strongly suspected a milk allergy, and noted that the problem was at its worst after macaroni and cheese. Since she had seen me go through my whole experience, one day she asked hesitantly if I could test Amy for milk. We did, and found out that she was somewhat weak for milk, very weak for some cheeses and not at all weak for others. The perfect solution in my opinion would have been for her mom to learn to test her, but she was not comfortable with that, so I did it. We tried something out on her, an allergy neutralization that will be discussed in detail in *Chapter 12,* and determined a way to prevent the reaction. Her mom used this successfully for some time, and eventually Amy seemed to outgrow the allergy, or food intolerance, whichever it technically was. In successive years when it came back, we tested again, and basically repeated the process for her. As I said before, it is not a crucial application of muscle testing, but ... why not?

Meanwhile, my sister had begun to use muscle testing in her psychiatric social work practice. Here is where muscle testing changed some young lives in fascinating ways. The following are a some true stories from her practice. The first of these brings up a common difficulty encountered by parents of teenagers.

The teenager who listened to her body,
not her mother:

Let's call her Jessa. She had always been a weak child, sickly, with digestive problems, stomach distress and constant diarrhea. Furthermore, her immune system was weak, and she had missed a great deal of school due to her frequent illness. When she first came in for counseling, she had circles under the eyes, she was low on energy, and had the usual stomach distresses. Years before, she had gone with her mother to see a doctor, and had been told she was lactose intolerant. However, her relationship with her mother was stormy, and she had been breaking her diet, seeing it as something her mother was trying to do to control her life. She did not want to listen to Mommy anymore. Since it was the mother who had come for counseling, it was suggested that she tell her daughter there was a way to find out about food sensitivity in a non-invasive way. After hearing about this very strange sounding technique, Jessa came in simply out of curiosity.

But she was not yet convinced, and still feeling somewhat controlled by her mother, she only brought a few items to test. She tested weak for the dairy products, and strong for candy. This was not the authoritarian response she had expected. Her interest piqued, she voluntarily made another appointment and brought five foods to test. She had just come from a fight with her mother and had run out of the house, but she came for the testing. That day she found out meat was okay, and to her surprise and delight, a certain brand of yogurt and a favorite frozen dessert were okay too. She made another appointment and began voluntarily modifying her diet. On her next visit, she brought everything she could think of. She had mixed results with breakfast cereals, found out to her amazement that potatoes were to be avoided, and tested all the things she generally ate for snacks. By now a good working relationship had been established and she continued for counseling. The next time she came for a session, she looked great - no stomach problems or circles under her eyes, energetic, and very happy. She had decided on her own, to control her diet. It was her own body telling her what to do, and not her mother or any other outside controlling force. Furthermore, her family relationships had improved. When one is feeling ill, daily life becomes a struggle, and she was no longer feeling ill.

It turned out that she was about to go off to college, and her strong motivation for finding out about foods was that she wanted to know how to stay well while she was away. She was ready to take responsibility and not lean on Mother. She even wanted to test to see which vitamins were good for her. This was a real turning point, since her mother had always wanted her to take vitamins for her health, and she had resented it. She became more hopeful and less frightened about going away to school, and had a wonderful lesson not only in food choices, but in her ability to take control of her life.

Teen alcoholism, addiction or allergy?

This was Jessa's sister, who came in for counseling after she was found guilty of DWI (driving while intoxicated) and had been mandated by the court to go for therapy. Although she had been an "A" student in high school, she had flunked out of college. It seems that she had started hanging out with a group who went out and drank beer, not all that unusual for college kids. But somehow for her, things would get out of hand. Once she started drinking beer, she found herself unable to stop. Was it an addiction? Was she just "letting herself go" for some reason?

And so, she had been court ordered to go to therapy. She had also learned about muscle testing while observing her sister, Jessa, progress in therapy, and she had watched with curiosity as Jessa's attitude brightened and allergies stopped ruling her life. During a discussion, Jessa had explained something that she had heard from her therapist (my sister) and which is often stated within the holistic community, namely, that when you crave something and yet eating it does not satisfy you, it may be a form of allergy. She knew that once she had started drinking beer, she was incapable of stopping.

Armed with this information, and basically an intelligent, sensible girl, she came to her therapy session with a can of beer and a bottle of wine. She muscle tested weak for the beer and strong for the wine. What did this result mean? To call it an "allergy" would be a slight stretch of the term. After all, she had no physical reaction to beer. Or did she? perhaps the craving was a form of intolerance we might just as well call an allergy.

She was not only amazed, but also reassured. Perhaps her drinking problem was a physical weakness. Maybe she wasn't a "bad kid" after all. This information must have also been a great relief to her mother. Even the potential solution was revealed by the testing. If she could stop having beer, maybe socially drink wine instead, with normal control, she could stop the cycle of trouble.

Since she only came in the one time, we do not have a detailed ending for this story, but the implications for us all are certainly noteworthy. A psychological dependency or an acting-out child can be helped by therapy, but perhaps there may be a physical response to a food that drives certain types of addictive behavior. Such information would be very valuable to anyone trying to help.

Camp food:

Max came in at age 16, having suffered from stomach problems his whole life. It had simply been accepted as fact, no particular testing had been done. He was a constant user of an antacid, and presumably had gotten to a state of medical semi-control. But now things had gotten out of hand. He had come home from camp to see a gastrointestinal specialist because of the severity of the diarrhea and stomach pains. He came to counseling before having the scheduled GI series. He was asked to bring in a sample of all the foods he craved and ate a lot of. He tested weak to milk, pizza, potatoes and chicken. Tomatoes and everything else he brought in was strong. It turned out that at camp, he had been eating a steady diet of pizza, chocolate milk, cheeseburgers and french fries.

After the visit, he went off the pizza and fries, and reported that he was feeling better, but not completely. We found out later he was still eating cheese, not realizing that the milk results would extend to cheeses. After the next session, he cut out the cheese too, and that was it. He felt all better and declared himself cured completely.

Holistic health in reverse:

This unusual situation involved a mother who was nutritionally very aware, and wanting to do the best for her child, she had taken him to a holistic MD and a nutritionist. Early on, they had been counseled to avoid dairy products. She followed diligently, and as a result, he had been deprived of many of the foods children usually eat. He had only been given soy milk, soy cheese etc. for years. Stomach distress had brought him to my sister's office for testing, and some unexpected surprises emerged. He tested perfectly strong for milk, but weak for soy! Imagine that, a mother who had worked so hard to modify a diet, and a child whose limitations in normal living had actually backfired. Who knows how long the child had been able to eat dairy and had not done so.

It would be presumptuous to assume the holistic doctor had been so terribly wrong from the beginning, so let us consider it another way. It is likely that after a long period without dairy, and with a high concentration of soy in his diet for the same long period of time, his original sensitivity to dairy was no longer there, and he had developed a sort of overdose effect to the soy. Again, muscle testing came in as a retesting device, to check for changes, in a similar way to my own situation when my mother regained strength to tomatoes. Again, the point came home to us that anyone who has ever been sensitive to any food should have this tool at their disposal, to keep a continuing eye on the progression of events. For this child, periodic retesting could have freed him up to live a more normal life and put an earlier end to the discomfort.

The previous stories are just a sampling of the effects of muscle testing I have been grateful to witness within a few short years. They all occurred through a snowball effect following my own difficulties and our fortunate rediscovery of the process. It is wonderful that some lives have already been changed for the better. But it is just a drop in the bucket, compared to the widespread good that can be done. I hope to show that anyone can learn to take control, change lives and spread miracles. In retrospect, it almost seems worth it to have gone through the temporary hell I did to find this little gem.

Chapter II

I am not allergic—Why would I want to know about muscle testing?

First let us agree on what we mean by allergic. In this book I use the term very loosely, not just in the formal medical sense of an IgA (immunoglobulin A) reaction. To us here, a food allergy will refer to any negative response after eating something. These could include exhaustion, jumpiness, nausea, aches, any stomach distress, localized throbbing, blotchiness, even irritation, hyperactivity, or depression, as well as the typical allergic responses of hives, breathing difficulties, and anaphylactic shock. Muscle testing can pick up any kind of weakness. If you ask your body, "Will this food cause a problem for me?," it will answer without needing you to get specific about the exact medical mechanism involved. Thank goodness for that.

However, if you ask an MD, you will find the first group of reactions mentioned above do not involve IgA, and therefore are called something else, perhaps an "intolerance" or a " sensitivity." To the sufferer, that does not do much good, and so we are not going to make those distinctions here. Therefore, when we call this chapter "I'm not allergic," we mean those people who really do not have negative reactions to foods.

So what could this chapter be about? By now you may already have some answers to this question, or could think of some, based on *Chapter One.* Let us look at ways in which everyone can benefit, and see why non-allergic people also need to know about muscle testing.

Will I react to the medicine?

In a nutshell, muscle testing can tell whether a new medication is safe to take. In *Chapter One* we saw that muscle testing enabled my mother to determine the safety of medicines before she took them, and the lack of it put her at severe risk. In my opinion that is one of the most important reasons everyone needs to know this technique. As for me, I have always been allergic to penicillin. As a child I remember when I took it and my lips blew up and turned bright red. Since then, penicillin has been out of bounds for me. But I found out the hard way, I had to go through that first reaction in order to find out about the allergy, just as everyone who is allergic to a medication does. Or maybe everyone does not have to go through it at all.

What about those people whose initial allergic response or side effect is severe or even dangerous? Do we really have to go through it to learn about such a sensitivity? My mother has had at least three severe reactions to new medication, because of a lack of prior knowledge. One was relatively minor, and involved stomach distress followed by a brief fainting spell during which she momentarily lost bowel control. It was scary, but a relatively minor reaction, which seemed to have no long lasting effect. The other two were much more serious, one being the prednisone-related tachycardia attack described in *Chapter One*, and the other being the disease called Bullous Pemphygoid, which emerged subsequently and in connection with hives after she took a particular pain killer. (At this point I must state that we have no "proof" that these two reactions definitely were caused by the medications, and that some doctors will discount any such relationship. Nevertheless, I and my family firmly believe these relationships are quite real.) Could these ordeals have been prevented?

We tried testing, after the fact, in all these cases. As for the prednisone, she tested weak as detailed previously. She also tested weak when we tried testing the drug that gave her the stomach distress. Months later, we tried a test of the same drug, and she was strong. We inferred from this that it may have been a buildup of the medicine in her blood that caused her to get to the point of the reaction, or at the time of the second testing, maybe her system was stronger and could have stomached it better. As for the pain-killer, we never did test her until months later, and at that time she also tested strong, so we do not have a real answer. But by now we all are convinced that she should have tested for all those medications before taking them and while taking them. You can bet she now insists on being tested before starting anything new.

Perhaps you can remember a time when you or someone you know suffered from some side effect or allergic reaction to a medication. Hopefully the consequences were not serious, but what if they had been? Muscle testing is the clear answer. By now, any new medication being started by anyone in my family is muscle tested. It is amazing to me that doctors do not use this tool routinely in their practices before prescribing anything strong. Maybe some day they will...

Adoptive Parents:

An addendum to the previous point. In the case of adoptive parents, they often do not have complete medical histories of the birth-parents, and are therefore deprived of some of the family information parents generally have in making decisions about their children's health. They are not able to say, "the stomach ache might be the peanuts, your uncle Frank is allergic to peanuts too" or "you have that same blotchiness your grandmother has when she eats citrus." These mothers and fathers would find an important and useful tool in muscle testing, to determine sensitivities or allergies not only to common items, but especially to medications.

Is the green food in the fridge safe?

Okay, I will admit it. I'm not such a great housekeeper. I also do not like to throw things out if they can be used. It used to be a joke in my house, in fact one friend will never let me forget the green meat—it had to get to that point before I finally gave up on it. After

I developed the food allergies, I had to become much more observant of the state of freshness of anything I was about to eat. This became especially true after an incident involving bread from a health food store that was a month late, (more about this in *Chapter III*) and caused me a week of suffering.

After that little incident, I realized I had better stop eating anything that might have any fermentation or mold, even invisibly, and that we would have to test anything in the refrigerator that had sat there for any amount of time. My husband, the thrower-out, has been totally vindicated. He is the one with the very sensitive taste buds—he can identify something that is not totally fresh long before I notice anything. In the past I used to brush off his refusal to eat this or that as "just picky," and I'd eat it myself. Since I used to have an iron stomach, I had no reaction, which convinced me further that he was just being picky. But now I have a new respect for his taste buds, and in more cases than I would like to admit, he has said, "This doesn't taste right, let's test it," and invariably I test weak for it. Nowadays that means it goes to the garbage immediately. In fact, due to my present set of weaknesses, I am used as the one for testing to see if there is anything wrong, because I will show the first sensitivity.

But my refrigerator is not the issue, yours is. I recall once hearing a comedian make a very funny routine out of the colors things turned in his refrigerator, and his inability to identify them after some time. I laughed a lot, and so did a lot of other people, I think because it hit home for more of us than we would admit. So, how about the idea of using muscle testing, not for the unidentifiable greenish brown thing that is headed for the garbage anyway, but for the perhaps slightly bad container of ricotta cheese that might cause some distress if it accidentally ended up in the lasagna?

All kidding aside, muscle testing really ought to be used on anything in our refrigerators that is at all questionable. In this society of relative prosperity, it makes no sense to eat something that will make us sick, even a little sick. And muscle testing can let you know in advance if it will.

Restaurant Dining —for better or worse:

Perhaps the very slow service should have been a warning that something was about to go awry. This restaurant was usually good, but when the Scampi finally showed up, we did the routine muscle test for me to make sure they really left out the lemon, as I had requested. No good, the arm went right down.

I groaned. We had waited so long for this dinner and I was really starved. "Why don't the cooks ever listen to me?" I wailed. I was at a severe allergy state then, and there was very little else on the menu I could have. What to do? While I pondered my lack of choice, Michael asked to be tested. "Oh, you and your weak stomach," I thought, and proceeded to push his arm down like a feather. Both amazed, we turned to my brother-in-law Julie, the third person who had ordered the Scampi. He is Mr. Iron Stomach-No Allergies, and yet his arm flew right down too. He bravely decided to try a taste, so we could all figure this out. He tasted...and spat. "Ech!" Shrimp went flying onto the table. Wow, this had suddenly become much more than a cook who did not listen to my dietary request. We gave back three dinners on the basis of his one bad taste. They were not happy. I suppose they would have liked us all to go through the tasting process on our own plates, but the muscle tests had made that unnecessary. I breathed a double sigh of relief that I had not taken a bite without testing.

Now let us look at a counterpoint to that story, an opposite situation in another restaurant. It was at least a year after the previous incident, and Michael had ordered salmon. He is not allergic to salmon and so no testing was necessary. However, when he took a bite he winced and hesitating, finally spat into his napkin. "Something's wrong with the fish, it's bitter - test me." I did and he tested strong. "Not unsafe, just not good," I responded. We tried me, just to make sure. If I test strong, it has got to be safe. I did, and even tasted it to confirm his opinion. I did not notice much of anything, maybe a slight bitterness, but I do not like salmon anyway. Anyway, this time muscle testing let us know it was okay for him to have the dish. Sometimes that is just as important as knowing when the food is bad.

Here is a fitting ending to this trilogy. Recently Michael went to a restaurant without me, and with Barbara and Julie and my Mom. My mother was the only one who did not order salmon. They said it tasted fairly good, but had some bitterness and they really did not enjoy it the way they had hoped. Later that night, and early the next morning, all three of them ended up running to the bathroom with a diarrhea attack, and Barbara and Michael felt odd the whole next day. No one had tested anything.

So, let us recap the message in this collection of true stories. First, if you are not allergic, muscle testing can tell you whether the food is bad, before or after you have tasted it. If you have possible sensitivities, maybe you do not consider yourself really weak, but you would just like to put your mind at ease, muscle testing can do that. In an ideal situation, we would all test everything, but that is unrealistic. Nevertheless, it is a valuable tool there for you to use whenever you want information.

Is overweight an allergic reaction?

My sister just could not get rid of those 10 pounds, no matter what she did. In late July 1996, she had read a local newspaper food column which discussed a study in the then current issue of the *American Journal of Bariatric Medicine*. In this study, 98 percent of people who eliminated foods to which they had tested allergic lost weight and body fat. According to the principal investigator, increased appetite and food cravings are some people's allergic-type reaction to certain foods.

Shortly after reading the column she asked me to test her for some foods she ate regularly. She runs and works out, and is generally so strong that I have difficulty getting a weak response from her even while she is holding poison. (No, that does not mean she can eat poison, it means I need to use one of the troubleshooting techniques discussed in *Chapter 5*.) Once we got a good weak and strong baseline, we tested. She was strong for everything, including wine, but when we tried bread she became totally weak. Was it wheat, a common allergen or possibly the yeast? No. The shredded wheat was okay. It was just the bread. As a result, she stopped eating bread for a couple of weeks. Five pounds slipped right off.

Now, let us think analytically. I would not base a theory or write a book that depended on this as sole proof of anything, or even write about it here, if it were not for the article in the medical journal. After all, it seems possible that she lost the weight because she ate less by cutting out bread. Or was it really a bit of an allergy? She did test weak, after all. But the next five pounds did not come right off. Was that weight a natural body plateau weight for her? Perhaps by eliminating an allergen her body was able to slide easily to a natural stopping point. This one needs more data before I am totally convinced. Nevertheless, since it is always a good idea to eliminate food items that test weak from anyone's diet, there is no reason not to try to lose a few pounds that way too. I'd be curious to hear the results.

Camping out, eating off the land:

We have come so far from the time when we all grew our own food and the norm was to live directly off the land, that it is sometimes difficult to believe that anything we can simply pick could be safe. I often wonder how ancient humans knew what was safe. Do you think they just ate randomly and died if a mistake was made? Is it possible they had some intuitive animal sense, perhaps could just "know" what was safe? Do you think they used muscle testing or some other intuitive ability? I wonder. It would answer some questions for me, to think a tool like that had possibly been in use eons ago.

Well, for us twentieth and twenty-first century people who would like to eat off the land, there is a simple answer. If muscle testing can identify shrimp that will make us sick, certainly it can identify berries or mushrooms that will make us sick. So muscle test away, and enjoy nature's fruits without danger or worry.

Vitamin Dosages:

Let us go back to 1978, when I first witnessed muscle testing as done by Don in New Jersey. We had gone to him because we were interested in improving general physical health and dealing with some minor problems. Don had gained a reputation as a healer of sorts, having helped numerous clients overcome various maladies, some serious, through a general strengthening of their bodies using vitamins, minerals, enzymes, and other holistic types of supplements.

His tool was muscle testing. He used a form of the "Applied Kinesiology" now done by many chiropractors to gain information about which parts of the body were weak, and then using the information about the body gained in this kinesiologic muscle testing, proceeded to test for forty or more possible food supplements. Our arms would go from strong to stronger to weaker, as he had us hold different numbers of vitamin capsules. Muscle testing determined the optimal dosage of everything as well as what we needed.

Every few weeks we would come back for retesting and adjustments in the amounts to take. During the time we were seeing him, we did feel better, more energetic, healthy, vibrant. But we eventually stopped because the trip to Jersey was just too much, and we often found ourselves taking thirty or more pills a day. We began to question it. I suppose the faith aspect needed was more than we could deal with, given the obstacles. Also, the nebulous nature of what was happening was not enough of a "proof" for us to continue.

Looking back, two strangely prophetic events took place then. First, Don kept telling me I should be doing the testing (MRT, he called it) myself, and that I really did not need him to do it. I could not accept this. I felt I needed some "teaching" and there was no way I could possibly do it the way he could. Secondly, he decided to lend me his basic book on muscle testing. I was curious enough to take it, and a year or more later realizing I had forgotten to return it, I called him. He said it was fine, he wanted me to have it anyway. And so I kept it. Some fifteen years later, when I was in the throes of horrible allergy and my sister and I rediscovered the idea of testing, that book was waiting on my basement bookshelf, to crystallize the old ideas, to reassure me, and to remind me what muscle testing could do.

Unfortunately, the book, entitled *MRT—Muscle Response Test*, by Fischmann and Grinims, 1978, went out of print years ago. The publisher told me no one believed it. I can understand why, since there was no clear black and white evidence it was definitely doing something, like the evidence I was given by my own allergies. Also, the book made many extravagant, but unsubstantiated claims, and did not focus on any one use of muscle testing, but rather sketchily implied it could be used for at least twenty esoteric purposes. But it was the book I needed in 1994, and for that I thank Don, wherever he may be.

The bottom line here is that you can use muscle testing anytime you would like to take a vitamin or food supplement, to determine an optimal dose. You will find that holding different quantities of it will make you weaker or stronger. To do this you will need to have a tester who has been at it long enough to have developed a feel for degrees of strength. This comes with practice. In any case, it is a perfectly good use of this quite versatile technique, for non-allergic situations.

Irritable bowel, hiatus hernia, etc:

There are certain conditions doctors can easily fix, and then there are other things that we often just learn to live with. The two mentioned here are digestive-type conditions with which I have had personal contact.

My friend Michele with irritable bowel syndrome "knows" she cannot ever have green or red peppers, but a variety of other foods are sometimes problematic and sometimes not. She never knows for sure what might trigger an attack, so she lives in a continuing state of insecurity. The couple of times I did dine with her, I was able to test and let her know what was safe for the time being. Curiously enough, the first time while trying several questionable foods she wanted to know about, she actually tested strong for peppers. But she was too afraid to even try eating them, after all, the whole idea of muscle testing does require a leap of faith. The other time, she tested weak for the peppers, confirming her basic knowledge and convincing me the first test was truly accurate for that time. Based on my findings, she limits herself more than she really has to.

She is a perfect example of someone who needs to have a spouse and/or child learn to test, so that she can have a constant reading on what is allowable at the moment, and relax while enjoying a maximum variety of foods. Unfortunately, her husband is basically a non-believer. One lesson I have learned is that when someone is ready to do this, they will do it, but it is useless to try to push it on someone who is not ready.

Michael's father, my father-in-law, was told he had a hiatus hernia. I recall he always used to be taking a certain antacid, and I know he pretty much ate whatever he wanted. I do not know what happened at night, but I do know he was somewhat of an insomniac. Now, when Michael would lie on his left side to sleep, he would often have a reflux response -- in other words, food would come up. He assumed he had some kind of situation similar to his father, but did not want to become a regular antacid drinker, so he stopped lying on that side, and the difficulty was no longer an issue. After we had started testing him for everything and he made the overall set of changes in his diet, some time later he told me he noticed he had no more difficulties lying in any position in bed. This was an interesting side benefit we might not have even noticed.

The doctors will probably want to "kill" me on this one — am I now saying that people with legitimate illness should not come to doctors to have them cured? I hope not. But on the other hand, there are some physical problems that might not be triggered if certain foods are eliminated, and if the person involved is willing to make that trade-off, why go through something like a surgical procedure? This paragraph is my disclaimer — I am not suggesting anyone neglect their proper medical care. However, I would love to see doctors using this kind of individual information to improve their personal care of patients.

To end this chapter, here is my wish list of all the types of people who, in my perfect world, would muscle test regularly as part of their profession:

Baby nurses: Yes, newborns can be tested by a surrogate method. This is a great way to see what milks or formulas they can safely tolerate, before they are given anything to drink.

Nutritionists: One of my sister's counseling clients found out the jar of vitamins given to her by her nutritionist was making her weak. She had been suspicious since she felt she was having a bad stomach reaction after taking them, and requested the testing. All she needed was another brand.

Geriatric Physicians: Since my mother's situation, I have heard too many horror stories about older people, especially in Florida, who have gone through dangerous scary ordeals and damaging side effects because of medications prescribed by their physicians. It would seem that the older metabolism might be easier to knock off balance by unfamiliar chemicals than younger bodies. If only physicians would test first.

Any Physician: In my "perfect world," why not give all patients the same security?

Personal Trainers: These professionals often suggest various protein powders and other supplements to aspiring body builders, as well as those who just want to look and feel stronger. These ought to be given the okay for each person, since often they push the limits of balance in giving mega amounts of one nutrient or another. It is just a safety precaution in this situation.

Psychotherapists: All the case studies from my sister's practice described in *Chapter One* should make it clear how useful muscle testing can be in dealing with larger emotional and family related problems. In this situation, testing would not be used on everyone, just on those clients whose problems cause a food related situation to become suspect. According to my sister, this happens more than we lay persons might realize.

I think we have described enough situations to make it clear that muscle testing can benefit everyone!

Chapter III

Is This "Scientific?"

The question has been asked of me many times, mostly at restaurants. The first time I heard it, I had a difficult time knowing what to answer. "What does it mean to be scientific?" I asked back. After all, this is not an officially endorsed medical method. It has not been the subject of statistical research studies. If I said "no," did that mean I was invalidating myself or saying I was doing witchcraft? What did this question really mean, anyway?

With all that confusion in my mind, I finally told Joe (not his real name) that I could not answer the question, but if he wanted to see simple proof that the technique truly worked, we could easily do that. He was obviously intrigued, and asked for the proof.

The search for decaf:

At that point in the evening, we were having dessert, six of us, and Michael and I had already stood up and down several times testing to see what would be safe for me to eat. In order to determine what desserts I might be able to have, we had to let everyone order and get theirs first. We had gotten good results on two dishes, including Joe's, and I suppose after he allowed me to hold his dessert he needed to do something in his own defense. I believe he felt silly even to have us at his table.

Anyway, feeling somewhat attacked but anxious to make my point, I told him to mix up the positions of our coffee cups, and we would tell him which was the decaf. Michael and I both turned our backs to the table, and our friends played the "shell game" with the coffee cups. Now, I normally test weak for caffeinated coffee and strong for decaffeinated, and Michael is exactly the opposite, so we could not only test me, but verify by double-checking him. When we turned around and saw the two identical cups, just for a moment I realized we were facing a challenge from potential skeptics, and a tension gripped me. Would we get it right?

Fortunately, I also realized that I no longer knew which cup was safe for me to drink, and that was more important than Joe's belief system. With that in mind, we quickly tested and found the decaf for me. Some of the group had already forgotten which cup was which, but my inquisitive friend verified that we had gotten it right. So long as I was focused on finding out what I really needed to know, the testing was smooth and easy. Would nervousness or a need to impress a skeptic have made the process less accurate? Maybe, maybe not, but later on, in *Chapter Five* on the method, we will see where attitude can make a difference.

At the time I hoped Joe was impressed. I was so thrilled with muscle testing that I felt a missionary zeal about convincing the world that everyone needed to learn it. Now I feel a bit differently. When people need to know something for their own benefit, they will be open and ready to accept the reality of muscle testing, and relieved to see that it does work. They will not likely ask if it is "scientific," because once you have experienced it, the question is no longer needed.

However, since that evening, I have come to two additional answers to the question, "Is this scientific?" As a mathematician/logician/scientist myself, I offer this story as a demonstration of *The Scientific Method* — you know, the method you learned about in high school science, the one that is formally used to prove theories.

The Scientific Method and the ricotta cheese mystery:

First let us get straight on how the "scientific method" works. Basically, one starts with a theory that seems to explain some data. In the case of finding, for example, the bacteria that causes a certain illness, the hypothesis or guess is made that a certain bacteria is the one. This guess might be made, perhaps because we find that bacteria present in those who have the illness, or because of other convincing evidence. Now, to complete the loop in a sense, to close out the scientific method, we would then introduce the bacteria to a healthy subject, and if the subject developed the illness in question, we would have *proof.*

By accident, I completed the same loop with my own allergies. I say "by accident" because I never would have eaten a food I tested weak to on purpose. No matter how much of a scientist I am, I am not that much of a masochist to expose myself to several days of skin torture just to prove a point I already knew anyway. But, back to the story:

One night my extended family decided to cook a Saturday night dinner together rather than go to a restaurant. Cooking had already become a challenging situation because of my many food limitations, but when we combined those with my mother's limitations and my husband's limitations and my sister's limitations, there was not much of a menu left. So we decided to make a simple pasta with vegetables, and anyone who wanted to could add something to their own portion. I decided to put in some ricotta cheese, which I had been eating without any ill effect.

A few minutes into the dish my nose started itching. Feeling very upset, I started to give the cooks the third degree, "Did someone put in any basil? Any bay leaf?" I accused. When it was determined that no problematic ingredient was in the mixture, we decided to test me for the whole pot. Sure enough, I was strong for the vegetables. Had the pasta gone bad? We tested me for the pasta, and again, I was strong. Now I started to panic. Was the muscle testing failing me? If I could not trust the testing, I was lost! My sister said we should test the ricotta cheese. I protested "No, that's not it. I just ate that yesterday and it was fine!" She finally convinced me to try it and my arm went right down. What a relief to know the testing was working after all, and the cheese was the offending food. But why? Just the day before it had been fine.

My sister tasted the cheese alone, something I had not done before adding it to my dinner. She reported that it was starting to turn. I smelled the container and realized it was no longer quite right. Of course, I was upset at having the hives beginning again, but by that time I knew about the effect of garlic in my particular situation, and took a few pills. That would abort most of the worst hives. This left me free to think about what had just happened.

We learned three important things that night. First, not to assume anything is definitely going to be completely safe unless we have tested it. Second, ricotta cheese has a short shelf life and must be sniffed before I eat it. Third, and here is the completion of the scientific method, that if I did eat a food that I was testing weak to, I would get the hives.

There were several other occasions that served to convince me that this was indeed a foolproof technique. In too many of them, the scientific method was again completed in a similar way, in that I suffered an attack of hives after accidentally eating something I tested weak for. There were also times muscle testing appeared to not be working, times I began to doubt its reliability. Thank goodness, in each of these instances it turned out I was wrong, not the test. A couple of these situations will serve as examples. While muscle testing appeared at first not to be working properly, it was later found to produce unexpected truths.

Times I doubted it:

Let us go back to the restaurant with the shrimp scampi. (Actually, I never did go back.) When I had ordered the dish, I had asked that they not put any lemon or wine into mine. Michael and Julie also ordered the scampi, without the restrictions. When dinner finally came, I was very anxious to have some, but I fortunately tested first, and got the weak result. My immediate thought was that they did not listen to my special requests in the kitchen. It would not have been the first time. However, as you likely recall from *Chapter 2*, both Michael and then strong Julie also tested weak. It was at that point that I began to doubt the muscle test. Why was everyone weak? Only when Julie tasted, and spit out the shrimp, did we realize that the shrimp had simply gone bad. No matter how much they worked that recipe to fit my needs, that dish would have given me hives.

As a side point, that night we learned two new things. First, that muscle testing had great potential use in determining whether food was still fresh, and second, that I was able to eat some cuts of steak. You see, previous to that time I had tested weak for steak and had given it up as an option. But that night, my mom's friend had ordered a club steak and in my hungry desperation, I tried testing it. When I got a positive result, he kindly offered to share it with me while we waited for a new dinner to be made. We shared two of them that evening, and I remained fine afterwards. Shortly thereafter, researching this further in the supermarket, I learned that somehow I was able to eat flank steak, and club steak. The reason why was still a mystery, but, who cared? And how could I have ever determined that kind of exact information for myself any other way?

On another occasion, I falsely accused my husband of poisoning me with a coffee ice cream soda. It was an evening I was working hard at home, grading papers, I believe, and really needed a break. He came home with my favorite treat; coffee ice cream soda, for us all. I was skeptical, after all I knew I could not have coffee with caffeine. What about that coffee syrup? But I did test strong to the cup, and so I proceeded to really indulge. The next morning I awoke with a miserable case of swollen red face.

I was totally crushed. How could this happen? I had tested everything I had eaten the night before. Had the ice cream soda been ever so slightly weak? Did we test correctly? Could I even trust this thing anymore? Days went by, and not only did I have to go through the pain of the physical reaction, I had also had my confidence in muscle testing shaken, and that was equally upsetting.

A couple of days thereafter, one of my friends was at my house to pick up her child after playing with my daughter. While she was here she asked me to check her out for peanut butter, something she had suspected was not so good for her. (By now, for better or for worse, my reputation had spread.)

In order to start off, I needed to get a feeling for her initial muscle strength. To establish a baseline strong response, I picked up something "healthful," a loaf of whole wheat bread from the health food store. She held it and I pressed on her other wrist. We expected a strong response, but instead she couldn't hold up her arm at all. In disbelief, we tried the bread on my husband, who also tested weak for it. What was wrong with this bread? The list of ingredients looked safe enough, and these were strong people. It did not look moldy or smell bad. Of course, we tested me next and I was very weak. But why? This mystery lasted another day, as I grabbed anyone who entered my house and forced them to hold the bread, and got negative response after negative response. Was the test going crazy?

It was not until the next day that I realized what the problem had been. The date on the wrapper was one month off! The day of the month was fine, only the month was wrong. And with bread from the health food store, there were no preservatives. I got a big apology, and a credit, from my health food storekeeper. I then realized that many apologies were due my poor husband, who had borne the brunt of my anger and who must have felt terribly guilty about the coffee ice cream soda that we thought made me sick. I would never have guessed to test the bread as it seemed safe. But sure enough, I had eaten it with my vealburger the night of the ice cream soda — two slices of it, too.

Once again, we learned some lessons from this experience. First, one has to test *everything* in order to be completely sure. Second, bread mold is a very long lasting allergen. As explained by my doctor friend, it stays in your body a long period of time, which was why I kept having hives for an entire week (about twice as long as usual). And third, I learned to stop doubting the testing process and to realize that if things were not going right, it was I who had made an error and not the testing.

Conclusion:

So after all these experiences, how do I wrap up the question, "Is this scientific?" Answers to this question lie in the results. It is hard to argue with the evidence.

My final response to this question has two parts:

1. I don't care if it is or it isn't "scientific." It just works. and ...
2. If you smack your thumb with a hammer, will you be in pain? Is that scientific? This is equally scientific.

And if someone isn't satisfied with those responses, perhaps they are not yet ready to learn about muscle testing.

Chapter IV

*Why Doesn't the World Already
Know About This?*

That is a good question. If muscle testing is so easy, so useful, and so available, why aren't all already doing it? I was as confounded by this question as you might be. But in considering possible answers, several reasons presented themselves, and after examining them, it became more plausible that this potentially wonderful technique could have been overlooked by the majority, especially in our present-day culture.

In short, the factors working against Muscle Testing include:

- Our Western approach to medicine and knowledge
- The prevailing cultural feeling about doctors and our bodies
- The technique seems to present no business or financial incentives for any particular group
- A reputation for un-dependability, which comes from an incomplete understanding of the technique.

But first let's realize that some of the world already does know about this methodology. There are chiropractors who use "applied kinesiology" (muscle testing used for diagnostic purposes) in their practices. There are holistic health professionals who are aware of the existence of muscle testing, if not completely informed in some cases, who use muscle testing in their practices for many of the same reasons you would want to. Nevertheless, the news has not spread like the wildfire I would have expected. Why?

Western culture and medicine — attitudes and paradigm shifts:

"What are you doing? Are you crazy?"
"You don't really believe in that stuff, do you?"
"Aaaaaah, come on!"

These things have all been said to me, and sometimes with venom, too. It is understandable because the dominant paradigms of our present culture make the above responses the sensible ones, when muscle testing is discussed or demonstrated. It is perfectly reasonable to not believe something when it does not fit the paradigms. But how many of us are even aware that we exist in paradigms, which can limit our understanding if they themselves are limited.

So what is a paradigm, and what does it have to do with me?

Let us say a paradigm is a way of looking at the world, like a set of glasses through which we see everything. If the glasses are tinted red, the world looks different and different assumptions would exist about color. If we clear the glasses, we may decide we have now got it all, but perhaps we would still be without peripheral vision. Paradigms can do that, convince us that we know it all, when in fact we are still missing something.

In his best-selling book, *The 7 Habits of Highly Effective People*, Stephen Covey discusses the power of paradigm shifting. The term "paradigm shift" was first introduced by Thomas Kuhn in his book, *The Structure of Scientific Revolutions*, and refers to a change in a basic way of thinking, essentially a change in the lens or filter through which we automatically look at things. Our perceptions change as the lens changes. For example, the change from Ptolemy's view that the Earth was at the center of the universe, to Copernicus' view that the sun was at the center, was a major paradigm shift. This shift enabled us suddenly to make easy sense of some previously very complicated astronomy. The orbits of planets around a central Sun became simple circles or ellipses, while the same motions were seen as tremendously complex "loop-de-loops," by the previous paradigm of Earth at the center.

But paradigm shifting is not easy. This particular paradigm shift was accompanied by a great deal of resistance and anger, as well as persecution of those who espoused it and attempted to prove its truth. Galileo was, in fact, a victim of powerful persecution, and suffered greatly during his later lifetime because his invention, the telescope, helped "prove" the new theory. At the time, too many people in high places, including the religious/political establishment, were entrenched in the previous way of thinking. Indeed, their lives, their power base would be badly undermined by such a shift. How many of them could afford to be open minded?

Looking back to those people of the past, what could they have thought of this new theory? It is easy to decide that the old "closed-minded establishment" were purposefully ignoring new truths to save their own hides. It is very simple to dismiss them as "old fashioned," not "modern and progressive" like our society is now. Maybe that is partially true, maybe not, but in either case there must have been plenty of people who honestly felt the new information was craziness — probably people who had not seen the proof first-hand. Those people, perhaps open-minded and well intentioned, were likely saying, "If this were true, wouldn't we have known it by now?" Or perhaps, "Our present belief system explains everything we need to know and it has been working fine. Why should we change?"

And what does this all have to do with us? At this point in time, as we enter the 21st century, we seem to be sufficiently technologically and scientifically advanced. Do we look back on Ptolemy as an under-informed primitive scientist, and Copernicus and Galileo as the ground-breakers of "real truth?" Does our present mastery of the three-dimensional world put us at an upper limit of knowledge? Could it be there are other things our scientific/medical system has not even considered? Is it possible that we are "dinosaurs" of a different sort? If so, could our culture endure a paradigm shift of a similar magnitude?

Consider the following paradigm shift:

In addition to what we can sense with the usual five senses, there exists an energy field around and outside the body. This energy field changes constantly according to the physical, emotional, and mental experiences of the person. It can be measured and used to obtain information. This new[1] concept underlies muscle testing and when used as a paradigm for understanding, makes the entire idea quite logical. Although the question of how muscle testing works will be discussed in *Chapter Six*, let us simply say at this time that a disruption in the energy field, caused by an offending substance placed within it, will weaken the body. Simple, isn't it?

However, such a paradigm does not exist at present for the majority of Westerners, and flies in the face of "traditional" Western medicine. I say "traditional" because there are an increasing number of medical doctors in the United States who are opening their minds and their research to the possibilities of energy fields; and I believe the 21st century will bring some changes.

So for now, people tend to respond to the possibility of muscle testing in a wide variety of personal ways. My experience has been that there are some people, who, when confronted with the reality of muscle testing, especially when demonstrated in undeniably accurate situations, become uneasy, upset, even hostile. Perhaps those people feel the comfortable rug of reality is being pulled out from under them by such a possibility. One night my sister and brother-in-law were having dinner with another couple who have been close friends for many years, and they began to muscle test each other before eating certain foods. Their friends were so antagonized by the entire concept that they almost got into a fight over it. Somehow relaxed discussion on the issue was totally impossible, and the evening could not even continue in a friendly way until the subject was dropped totally.

1 - Not so new really—the use of the body's energy field has been common practice in Chinese Medicine for thousands of years.

Others begin to giggle about the apparent flakiness of the situation, and dismiss the possibility immediately. One day a five year old friend of my daughter was at my house, complaining of the "itchies." My daughter Melinda confirmed that her friend had been having hives on and off for quite a while. She said her mother told her she could not have any milk (among other foods). Curious, I tested her, and found out she was perfectly strong for milk, but very weak for American cheese. When I presented this information to her mother and volunteered to go to the supermarket with them for a full testing, she began to laugh loudly said, "Get outta here!" gave me a friendly poke in the shoulder and refused to hear any more about it. Her daughter remained on a very restricted diet given to her by an allergist for an extended period of time. So unfortunate, so unnecessary, but be ready to live with frustration if you become involved in muscle testing. Some others just become detached and bored, shrugging it off as something they would rather not waste time discussing.

It can be unsettling to witness proof that an energy field surrounding the body exists, and even stranger, that it could be actively used to make important decisions. Perhaps it is scary to think that we really do not know it all, that some fundamental solid belief systems are not so solid. Our present Western world paradigm, and indeed, the paradigm that underlies all Western medicine, completely ignores the existence of energy fields surrounding the body.

So in sum, people will feel threatened, even insulted. They will dismiss it as crazy and laugh it off. Furthermore, and here comes the *Catch 22*, if we attempt to do muscle testing on a person who harbors negative feelings, expressed or unexpressed, to force proof on them, chances are it will not work. Boy, will you feel silly then! (This twist will be discussed more fully in *Chapter 5* on the method, and *Chapter 10* on *Sabotaging the Results*.)

Fortunately, if you are doing muscle testing in order to obtain information, it will be clear in such cases that the testing is not working, right from the start, so there is no danger of getting incorrect information. But the fact is, those who deeply do not want to believe this can work will feel justified when the method fails for them. That is exactly what happened when I naively ran to my pediatrician, a lovely older gentleman and a good friend, with my thrilling new discovery, and I tried to show him the technique before I completely understood its idiosyncrasies. Nothing worked. I could not even get started. Boy, did I end up feeling like a fool. I probably would have given it all up as unreliable, had I not been totally dependent upon using muscle testing then and for years thereafter, and gotten consistently accurate information.

So where does this all leave us? If we shift our paradigm to allow for the existence of a real, measurable, usable energy field around the human body, something like muscle testing becomes quite reasonable and logical. If we see it through the lens of the prevailing Western cultural view, it seems like impossibility, flakiness, wish-fulfillment or many of the other epithets with which it has been dismissed in the past.

Our feeling about our bodies and our doctors:

Let us take a look at the way we, in Western society, tend to use doctors. We are socialized to "trust the doctor" implicitly because they have superior knowledge. That can be very useful in allaying our feelings of fear when we are ill. The fact that someone really knows what is best for us and can "cure" us, is immensely powerful and appealing. More and more, as the medical community has become increasingly specialized and scientific research has progressed, we are in awe of the results. And this feeling is appropriate. It is truly amazing what modern medicine has accomplished, from life support, which saves lives, to reproductive technology, which creates lives, to microsurgery and so many other miracles which have been performed. These are wonderfully positive additions to our life.

The flip side of this very positive gift to humanity is what has happened to us as individuals. In a way we have given away power, we have become weaker. It is intimidating, even scary, to do something "medical" for ourselves. It is sometimes easier to take a pill than make a decision. For me, I had to get to the point of giving up on the medical establishment because they really could not help me, before I searched for and discovered other alternatives. Many people are uncomfortable with the idea of taking health issues into their own hands. And that makes it much harder for something like muscle testing to become accepted into the mainstream.

To use Muscle Testing to determine food intolerance, is to say to yourself, "I am ready to take control, and responsibility, in this situation. I am not going to relax and let some higher authority to do it for me." And even more powerfully, "I am able to do something that is as effective, or maybe even more effective, than a medical test." That can be pretty intimidating. One has to get beyond that feeling of intimidation. And believe me, you do get beyond it. You get beyond it when you start to see how easy and reliable the results are. You get beyond it when you've tried it umpteen times and see it works consistently on foods you know about. Mostly, you get beyond it when you *need* to.

It isn't good business for anyone:

Who then, would want to spread the word? Who would be an advocate for muscle testing? As we know, many millions of dollars are spent each year on medical research involving new drugs. Drug companies spend much of this money for obvious financial reasons, and stand to gain everything by proving the effectiveness of their discoveries. Certainly no one in that area would be interested in financing research on muscle testing.

The medical profession certainly has no interest in investigating muscle testing, for many of the reasons mentioned above. There have been a handful of M.D.'s who have attempted to bring muscle testing to their colleagues, most notably John Diamond, M.D., who has been the most successful in spreading the word to medical professionals, including physicians and dentists. His books, *Your Body Doesn't Lie*, and *Life Energy*, have also reached a significant portion of the public, using muscle testing (also known as kinesiology, when used in certain diagnostic ways by medical professionals) as a basic method for getting information. But unfortunately, doctors like Dr. Diamond are few and far between, and often those who are brave enough to take these practices seriously, risk professional disapproval.

According to an article in *Life* magazine called *The Healing Revolution*[2], there is even a *National Council Against Health Fraud*, which includes doctors who openly dismiss thousands of years of Chinese medicine as crazy, homeopathy as not even worth testing, and who fervently believe that doctors drawn into those areas should lose their licenses. According to reporter George Colt, who wrote the article, *The American Medical Association* publishes a *Reader's Guide to Alternative Health Methods*, subtitled *"An analysis of more than 1,000 reports on unproven, disproven, controversial, fraudulent, quack, and/or otherwise questionable approaches to solving health problems."* This publication is sponsored by some of the same doctors in the *National Council Against Health Fraud*. When the *Life Magazine* reporters looked at the above mentioned *Reader's Guide* they found the word quack was used over 200 times in the first 36 pages. Just the subtitle of this publication, and that one figure, are enough for us to guess how something like muscle testing would be received by this group. Fortunately, according to the article, there are also an increasing number of medical doctors who are "coming out of the closet" regarding their beliefs, who have had experience with alternative therapies and are interested. But they are discouraged from or perhaps even afraid to pursue those interests. Who could blame them?

2 - September 1996 issue of *Life Magazine*, page 42

Nevertheless, I personally feel that the tide is changing, even in the medical world. As planet Earth becomes a smaller place, elements of Eastern thinking are being more and more heard and accepted in the West. Alternative therapies are becoming more a part of the norm, and more than ever widely used by the American public. The medical profession now includes more doctors than ever before who will admit the possibility of new frontiers that have not been explored, and I believe that the forthcoming generation of practitioners will begin to take very seriously some possibilities that twentieth century medicine has ignored.

Professionals who do use muscle testing :

There are actually several groups of professionals who already use muscle testing in their practices. In the 1950's, Dr. George Goodheart, a chiropractor, developed the science of muscle testing called *Applied Kinesiology*, which diagnoses weaknesses in various parts of the body. His work has been incorporated into the chiropractic curriculum, and Applied Kinesiology is now used diagnostically by large numbers of chiropractors in their practices today. Holistic practitioners incorporate forms of muscle testing into their practices for a variety of purposes. However, even for those who believe in and use muscle testing professionally, they do not generally promote muscle testing for the lay person. Many of these professionals feel Kinesiology is something to be done by Kinesiologists, and do not suggest their patients try it themselves, or attempt to teach them how.

In fact there has already been an entire book dedicated to the marvels of muscle testing. The previously mentioned book called *M.R.T. (Muscle Response Testing)* was written in 1978 by Drs. Fischmann and Grinims, a chiropractor and Oriental medical doctor, respectively. The book was a fascinating and fun source of complete information about the technique, and was intended for the lay audience. Fortunately, it sat in my basement for sixteen years and was there for me when I needed it. But it is now out of print, because, as the publisher explained to me, "no one believed it." It is my belief that this book, though excellent, had no way of proving in a black and white way that the technique could produce concrete results and fill a concrete need, and therefore never found its audience.

"Undependable"—inaccuracies and incomplete information:

One day I was discussing my allergies and my wonderful solution with the mother of a friend. She is a holistic nutritionist, and what I would call a "new-age person." When she found I was using "kinesiology," she said, "that's useful sometimes, but it really isn't dependable." At the time I did not understand what she meant, and I insisted that it was totally dependable for me. She said something about needing to be "neutral," which I largely ignored because I did not understand what she meant. It took me some time to understand her statement. But when I later encountered the need for neutrality, rather than causing me to dismiss the process as unreliable, it suggested ways of controlling the process for reliability.

Her response is typical of many who know about kinesiology. There are a lot of people who know a little about muscle testing, but very few who know enough to control all the possible errors and make it really work accurately. Even the literature by prominent holistic health professionals is full of semi-accurate methodology. For example, a well-known public speaker and health advocate stated in one of his books, that to test food by kinesiology, the food had to be put in the mouth. This twist on the method is unnecessarily cumbersome and dangerous for people with severe allergies. Another states that the method is not totally dependable, and suggests "playing" with it at home.

In *Chapter 5*, we will be discussing troubleshooting. There are certainly ways in which muscle testing can go wrong, if the tester is unaware of the delicate nature of an energy field. It was my own experience with clearly false results, which caused me to seek a deeper understanding and to learn how to control for the possibility of inaccuracy. Fortunately, anyone who does muscle testing can easily make sure it is working accurately. In *Chapter 10*, we will take a good look at ways of sabotaging the results. It is true that an unscrupulous tester, or someone who is not aware of all the in and outs, can create false results. This fact provides yet another reason that the testing you can trust the most is your own.

Chapter V

Directions for Testing

We have had enough introductory information. This chapter will cover several methods for muscle testing. The "basic" arm method is the one I have used repeatedly and successfully since 1994 in thousands of successful tests. I find it to be easiest to do, giving maximum control and precision of results. However, there are situations in which the basic method is uncomfortable, perhaps embarrassing or even not possible. For these situations you may use alternate methods that work perfectly well. Also we will discuss troubleshooting methods to be used when problems are encountered, and ways to control for inaccuracy. If the testing is not working accurately, you will know about it in advance, and therefore you need never worry about being misled by your results.

The best way to use this chapter is to pre-read it and get an idea of what will be happening, before trying anything. First read all of the information and troubleshooting hints and look at the illustrations to be sure you have the picture. Then, you will be ready to actually try it out step by step with your testing partner. Here we go!

The Basic (Arm) Method: It takes two, the tester, and the subject or person to be tested. The tester may be behind the subject, or the tester and subject may face each other. (Position is discussed more in *Troubleshooting* below.)

For the subject: Extend your arm out sideways, straight out from the shoulder and hold it up at an angle a little above 90 degrees. Find that comfortable "shelf"—that easy muscle lock that hangs the arm up. At this height, it will feel like your arm is relaxed or resting. Keep the wrist and hand straight out, not limp and hanging. Think about your arm, as if it were up on a shelf—the tester will now find that shelf by giving a firm but gradual press. Do not fight the pressure by pushing the arm upward, just keep it stable, relaxed and resist the downward pressure when it comes. Keep the arm where it is. Meanwhile, the other hand is resting on your stomach.*

For the tester: Generally speaking, you will be feeling for that shelf of muscle strength by pressing on the outstretched arm.

Stabilize yourselves by placing a hand on the subject's shoulder of the arm not raised. Then raise your other arm to gently touch the wrist of the subject's outstretched arm. ("Shall we dance?") Do not lean or press on the raised arm at all, a common error which can exhaust the subject. Warn the subject, by saying something like, "Ready?...Resist!" Then press firmly, but not suddenly, and try to find that shelf that holds the arm up. Of course you could press so hard that the arm comes down, but that is not the idea. You want to feel for that "shelf," that comfortable stopping point, where the arm becomes firm. This should only need to be done once. Everyone should stay fresh and comfortable, no one should become exhausted or muscle strained.

And that is the basic test. What you have just done is a test of baseline muscle strength. You now have a feel for the subject's strength in general. Now you need to do a baseline test for weakness. That will be an exact repeat, but with the subject holding something poisonous, like bug spray, against the

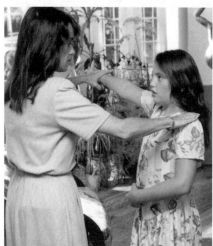

Basic Arm Method - *testing a child (tester may sit to test smaller child)*

stomach. (I have found that a little bottle of Jet Dry weakens everyone and is conveniently small and light.) If you can feel the outstretched arm go down when the poison is held against the stomach and stay up with an empty hand on the stomach, you can go ahead and test that person for anything.

Once both people know what "strong" feels like, and what "weak" feels like, accurate testing of any substance is done by feeling whether the muscle is weak or strong when the questionable substance is held

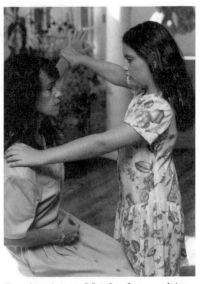

Basic Arm Method - *subject seated / child as tester*

in the subject's hand resting against the stomach. The tester will notice whether there is a weaker shelf or the shelf has disappeared completely, leaving the outstretched arm to buckle, or even to topple the subject with the same amount of pressure as in the strength baseline. Furthermore, the amount of weakness in the arm indicates the amount of weakness for that substance. When I was in my highly allergic mode, my muscle disappeared completely. It felt so strange to suddenly have my arm drop, as if I were not ready for the push. But a repeat of the strength baseline and the test reassured me the results were real.

An alternate method is available for determining a weakness baseline, in case you do no t have any poison available. I generally do not use it in my presentations to groups, because it looks strange and tends to cloud the "black and white"-ness of testing. But it is simple and it works. To get a weakness baseline, the tester will, instead of putting the free hand on the subject's shoulder, use that hand to poke the subject in the hollow of the cheek on that side.

Hold the finger with pressure into the hollow of the subject's cheek, and they will lose muscle strength in the opposite arm, giving you your weakness baseline when pushed.

Troubleshooting:

Bouncing arms: Hopefully during the strength baseline test you both felt a firm muscle lock, and things did not become bumpy or bouncy. Bumps and bounces are an indication that the testing is not clear or accurate. Before testing for a food or substance, both the tester and subject really need to get the firm baseline feeling, so let us eliminate the bounces. Bouncing often occurs when the tester comes down too suddenly or too hard or when the subject is "fighting." If you are getting bumps or bounces, try pressing less hard and/or less suddenly. Ease into it, and increase pressure till you both sense that point of stability. This should take at most two seconds. When you feel the stability, do not press any harder. Remember, this is not a con-test, but a cooperative effort by you both to feel a comfortable point of resistance. If anyone is getting tired or hurt, the push was too hard.

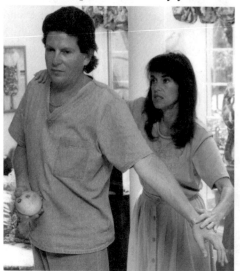

Positions and the sex factor: No, this title is not here to keep your interest. It is something that I am not at all happy with, but seems to be true nevertheless. It seems that when a woman and a man face each other, the woman tests weaker than usual and the man tests stronger than usual. Why this is true, whether it is innate

Basic Arm Method - *Opposite sex testing (subject is allergic to the onion)*

energy fields or learned by socialization, are perplexing questions, which could produce some fascinating and productive research. As for the technique, this factor can produce inaccurate results, and yet I have never seen it dealt with in any of the present literature for the public.

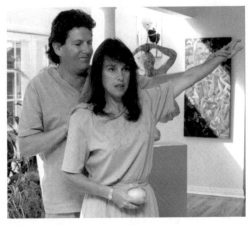

Basic Arm Method—Opposite sex testing

The solution is simple enough. Testing can always be done either face to face, or with the tester behind the subject. Notice that the directions above did not specify which position to use. Same sex testing may be done face to face. Opposite sex testing is better done with the tester behind the subject. If that poses a problem, the tester can always try to stand a bit to the side or face diagonally away while testing. It is the face to face position that causes the difficulty.

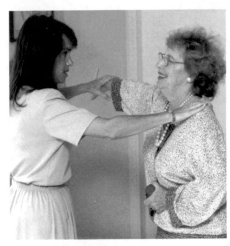

Basic Arm Method—Same sex testing

Before I knew about this situation, I noticed that it was generally harder to get the weakness baseline for males, and also that females tended to tire when tested by their husbands. When I do lectures and demonstrations, I generally have a husky man come up and "challenge" me to demonstrate the technique on him. I seat him and test from behind. It is amazing and often amusing for the group to see me, a relatively short and small boned woman, push down his arm easily in the weakness baseline, after I literally could not budge it in the strength baseline.

Accidental Short Circuiting: This a quirky situation that rarely ever happens. But to be totally prepared, you ought to know about it. If your subject just happens to be pressing his or her tongue against the roof of the mouth where it meets the teeth, the muscle testing will produce false strong results, no matter what is held against the stomach. A colleague of mine noted that that mouth position is spontaneously done when a karate fighter is about to strike, and yells one of those "Haiyaa!" sounds.

Subject too strong or too weak: It can happen. Someone you are trying to test can be so strong that their arm stays up, even when holding poison. It happened to me with my sister who is certainly no muscle man although she does work out regularly. This case is interesting because generally I can test her with no trouble at all. But one day she came back from jogging, and wanted to check on bread, something that usually weakens her. She tested surprisingly strong for the bread. I was suspicious. I tried to get a weakness baseline and could not. She actually tested strong for a can of bug spray. What was happening?

Muscle testing is an energy phenomenon. We have already said that and we will go into it in more detail in *Chapter 6*. What had happened was that her energy field was so strong after her morning run (she calls it her meditation, and seems to be glowing when she comes back), that it stayed strong enough to hold her arm up, even with poison or a poke in the opposite cheek.

The solution once again is an easy one. If you cannot get a weak muscle while holding poison, stroke the arm in the direction opposite to natural energy flow. That is, to temporarily weaken the muscle, stroke the subject's arm upward, from the tops of the fingers upward to the top of the shoulder. Do this three or four times, then repeat the test and you will find your weakness baseline. Test for questionable foods right away because the weakening effect lasts long enough to do some testing, but not more than a few minutes (varying time periods for different people). To be sure, redo your weakness baseline after doing the last test, to ensure it is still working.

To finish the story, I weakened her, got the baselines confirmed, and then found that bread was still not good for her. Now here is a case that cautions us all not to assume anything, and to always start with both baselines, even if we think we know someone's strength very well. The opposite situation can also occur: It happened with my mother, who was fighting off a skin disease at the time, and was generally weak. I could not get a baseline for strength. I tried and tried to feel the baseline muscle lock, the shelf, but it was mushy. With my most careful easing into the pressure, the shelf was still hard to find. Can you figure out what to do? Yes — just stroke the arm in the direction of the energy flow to temporarily strengthen the muscle. That is, stroke from the top of the shoulder downward to the tops of the fingers, three or four times. It works. Again the proviso, the strengthening effect lasts a few minutes, so double check your baselines as you go and at the end of testing.

Expectation can cause false negatives: This situation is discussed several times in this book because it is so important in the quest to make muscle testing totally accurate and trustable. I refer back to my daughter and her processed chips. I disliked the idea of her eating all that MSG and other chemicals, and was quite convinced it could not be any good for her. When she did indeed test weak for them, I was vindicated. I had her convinced too. But it was a lie. And that is the solid truth — your own negative expectation can and will cause a weak test.

Subsequently, after I learned about this situation, I retested her for the chips, this time fairly, and found to my consternation that she was perfectly strong for them. But after thinking about it for a while, for muscle testing to be a valid diagnostic tool, you do not want it to show a weak result unless there is really going to be a problem. So maybe it is just as well.

Okay, so how do you control your expectations? That question can be answered individually. When I test, I take my mind off what is being tested, generally peer off into space and just concentrate on finding that shelf. It works for me and many others. Some of my students envision a question mark while testing. Others will say to themselves "let's find that shelf," while doing the pressing, which focuses attention on the neutral concept. Fortunately, testing works best when you need it the most — when you really don't know what you can or cannot have, and you desperately want information.

Negative Attitude: This is a issue related to the previous one, but a bit nastier. Let us face it, there are people who really do not want to know that muscle testing can be for real. We have gone into that fact elsewhere in this book and we do not need to beat it to death here. I include in this group some dedicated MD physicians whose entire life's purpose and livelihood is threatened by the concept of an energy paradigm. How can an allergist be happy knowing that what they have studied a lifetime for and built their success and self-esteem on, can be easily put aside by you or me, as we get results without delay, without pain, and with at least as good accuracy. It takes a very very big person to be able to accept that without hostility. Even outside the medical fields, there are many people who become upset, hostile, even pugnacious when muscle testing or energy medicine is even mentioned.

If you try to test these people, you will get troubled results. The most common of these is the bounce mentioned earlier. You will bounce during the strength baseline. You will bounce during the weakness baseline, and you will not get the weakness. It will become a muscle competition. You will get tired. Give up. That person cannot and will not be tested, even if they have a smile on their face and seem to be amenable. There are some people who are just not ready to accept this. Don't knock your head against the wall trying to convince someone who is not ready to know. You will just exhaust yourself, and it will not work anyway. Give it time and send your positive energy to that person in your thoughts. Maybe next year.

Alternate testing methods for special situations:

Here are several other ways of testing. Although I have not used them as often as the basic method and I have had varying degrees of success with them, the protocol below will always ensure you get accurate results or no results at all. The rules to remember when doing any kind of muscle testing are these:

1. Get a clear baseline for strength
2. Get a clear baseline for weakness
3. Test the questionable items
4. If any test is unsure, repeat strength and weakness base lines to re-establish the "feel."

This protocol is your insurance for accurate results. If any type of testing is not working accurately and reliably, you will know it because the baselines will fail. If your baselines are clear and provide an obvious difference in the feel of the strength, your testing will be accurate.

Hand Method: This one is useful when you do not want to look conspicuous. I know people who will only do it this way when they are in restaurants, so that they do not get any weird stares. I personally do not mind the weird stares. I find them amusing and an opportunity to discuss the usefulness of muscle testing with strangers; but I can understand those who do not want to do that. So here it is:

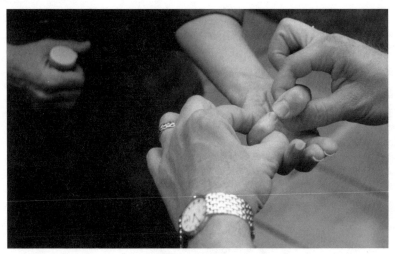

Hand Method - *discreet, done seated in restaurants*

The subject places the tips of thumb and pinky together (same hand), pressing fairly firmly to connect them in a sort of "O" shape. (See illustration.) The tester takes both index fingers, loops them into the "O", one finger on each side, and pulls, as if to open up the subject's "O." The tester is really finding the firm lock that keeps the fingers together, and gauging the amount of pressure just before the fingers would start to budge. The subject's other hand is on their stomach, as usual. This is the strength baseline. In the weakness baseline, the subject holds the poison against the stomach as usual, or pokes their own opposite cheek with the available hand. The "O" should pull apart with the same pressure that was used previously.

I have a friend who prefers this method to the basic arm method completely, and claims she has complete accuracy with it. It is truly a matter of preference, but again, the important thing is to ensure accuracy by getting a solid strong and weak baseline before doing your testing.

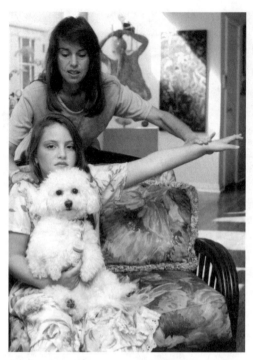

Surrogate Testing: In surrogate testing, you can become the substitute, or surrogate, for the subject. You connect up with the actual subject, as described below, and your own outstretched arm is used for the strength tests.

The first of these is most useful for babies and animals who will sit in your lap. It is quite simple. You sit down, seat the child or animal in your lap and you become the surrogate subject. Your outstretched arm is

Surrogate Testing - *on the lap for babies or small animals*

used in the usual way, and the hand that is usually on your stomach is now against the baby's or animal's stomach in front of you. Foods to be tested will be held in your hand against the child's stomach, baselines are done as usual and results obtained in the usual way. However, there is one important factor to consider. Any allergy or weakness you may have will be reflected in the testing along with any weakness the child or animal has.

For example, my sister wanted to check her infant grandson for pineapples. He had been getting some skin rashes and she was suspicious. We tried surrogate testing and he did test weak. Somehow he got hold of some pineapple anyway, and it had no ill effect. Was the testing wrong? We puzzled about this. Sometime later my sister was eating pineapple and her throat started to itch. Next time

I saw her we tested for pineapple and she was quite weak. It was then we realized what must have happened with little Adam. So be aware of that possibility, and then go ahead with confidence. Strong tests are real, in any case, taking place only when both of you being tested are strong.

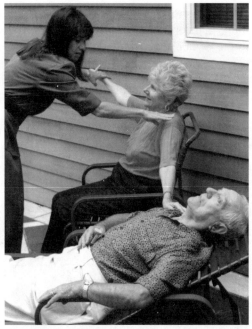

Surrogate Testing - *surrogate connects to subject's shoulder while subject is reclining (note pillbox on subject's stomach is being tested)*

The other surrogate test is most useful for someone who is perhaps confined to bed or a wheelchair and cannot cooperate with seated muscle testing by the arm method. This one is quite amazing, even to me. The way you, the surrogate, connect up with the actual subject is by outstretching your arm and resting your hand on the subject's shoulder. Then a food or substance to be tested is placed against the subject's stomach, either by them or a helper, and your remaining arm can be raised for the strength tests. I cannot personally vouch for this test in the same way as for the basic test, because again I have only found need for this test on a few occasions. However, I have gotten useful and accurate results on those occasions.

Self-testing method: Before concluding this section on alternate methods, I feel it is my responsibility to describe a self-testing method that has been shown to me by friends. I have personally tried this method several times and cannot get it to work reliably, but that does not mean it is without merit, and it is certainly something you can attempt. You form an "O" with the thumb and index finger of one hand. Then use the index finger of the other hand to try and pull through the two joined fingers, forcing them apart. That is the strength test. A strength baseline would be the amount of pressure that they withstand without separating. The weakness baseline is gotten by placing a poison in the palm of the hand that is forming the "O". The same amount of pressure from the finger attempting to separate the "O" should now pull right through. Test by putting small amounts in the palm of the hand.

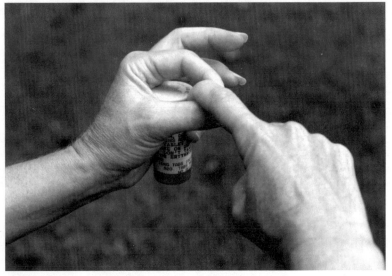

Self Testing with hands

What else do I need to know?

This is perhaps the most important bit of advice in this entire chapter. It is about patience and perseverance. Doing muscle testing is a bit like learning to ride a bike. There is a "feel" that one gets, a subtle knowing that comes across at a certain point, that suddenly enables you to get it right. Some people seem to pick it up immediately.

The first time they try to test, they get clear firm baselines and results. Others just do not. It is not a question of intelligence, or open-mindedness, or even of desire to learn. I have yet to find a pattern that can be used in predicting whether someone will pick this up more quickly or slowly.

In my own personal situation, I was very fortunate because my sister was an instant tester. No one taught her how to do it or led her through a testing experience by physically getting behind her and showing her how the pressure feels. She was accurate the first time, and thereafter. On the contrary, my husband took several weeks before we knew we could trust his results. During that time, when he tried to test me, it felt too strong, sometimes too weak, not firm enough or otherwise uncomfortable. The baselines did not feel comfortable, and the weakness baseline especially did not come through. My daughter, who was seven when she learned to test, picked it up within a couple of weeks of occasional trying, and her tests were perfectly accurate even at that age.

It is important for you to realize, as you begin your adventure into this realm, that it may not work right away, and that is perfectly okay. Do not give up and say, "muscle testing doesn't really work," as some have done in the past. It does work and it will work. It is as real as riding a bike is real. If you want to learn to use it, if you need to use it, you **will** learn. Just keep trying for those baselines, maybe a few times every day or two, and you will eventually get that feel. And once you have it, it is yours for good.

Chapter VI

How does it work?

In *Chapter 4* we spoke briefly about paradigm-shifting, and the fact that mainstream Western thinking does not include a "personal energy field" paradigm -- at least not yet. We also said that when one accepts the reality of an energy field surrounding the body, it becomes very easy and logical to discuss muscle testing. Let's get just a bit more specific here, using the same ideas.

Picture this:

There is an energy field surrounding the body, that is made up of circuits, not unlike the circuits that wire your house for electricity. Along one of these circuits in your house may be some lights, some appliances, perhaps a television. Have you ever blown a fuse or tripped the circuit breaker, and had a whole group of electrical items lose power at once? That is how it works with a circuit, or energy pathway like electricity. When one part of it gets into trouble, the entire circuit is affected.

Now let us think of our bodies in a similar way. Eastern philosophy and medicine describes a vast and complex energy system surrounding the body, that can be viewed as a series of energy meridians (circuits). This logic is at the basis of acupuncture, homeopathy, foot reflexology and a large variety of energy therapies that are becoming more and more commonly accepted, although they cannot be "explained" by Western medicine. If we short-circuit one of these meridians, the entire meridian of energy flow weakens.

As for muscle testing, let us envision a line of energy that passes along the deltoid muscles that lift the arms, goes around the fingers, along the muscles that lift the legs, the stomach area many would refer to as the "gut," and several other parts of the body. When someone holds a food or substance that is bad for them in this line of energy, all the muscles along that meridian weaken. Muscle testing becomes perfectly simple common sense, when looked at within the energy paradigm. Since the energy field extends a few inches around the body, there is an area within which we can place the offending substance, and it will affect the meridian, even if it is not inside or even touching our body.

And so, you can go to the supermarket, place a can or jar of tomatoes against the stomach, and get a weak result in muscle testing, even though the jar or can is still sealed shut. You can move a plate of food close to your stomach in a restaurant, and test to see if that food will hurt you, without getting sauce on your clothing. And no, you do not, as many have stated in other books, have to put anything in your mouth or even against your skin, in order to test it. (Thank heavens for that!)

Now let us look at your situation as a tester. If you begin to do muscle testing for those around you, there will undoubtedly come times when you will be asked to explain this strange looking process, and to justify it in some way. Let's equip you properly to answer and inform others, and to not be intimidated by arguments that might be presented.

I am basically a scientist and a logician. The explanation above makes sense to me, and hopefully, it will for you. It is simple, logical and explains the process. However, I have read in other literature about the subconscious, about body memory, instinct, the 85% of our brain we do not use, inner animal body wisdom and other explanations for the accuracy of kinesiologic types of muscle testing. I am open-minded enough to allow for the possible reality of all these. Rather than answering "how" muscle testing works so accurately, these types of explanations seem to be answering "why" it works. "Why" indeed does the energy field weaken when an offending substance enters it? That is more of a metaphysical question or even a spiritual one, and will involve belief systems belonging to the individual. I certainly would not attempt to answer it here.

So, be aware of the subtle difference between the questions, "How does it work?" and "Why does it work?" Realize that you can easily explain how it works, but if you are drawn into an argument or debate on metaphysical realities, it becomes a "why" question, and ideas become a matter of faith or opinion. Enjoy the debate, and understand that whatever is said in that context does not threaten your simple common sense, logical explanation of how muscle testing works.

Chapter VII

What Do the Results Mean?

There is no quick answer to this question. The fact is that testing will give different types of information for each person. The only thing we can say for sure is that a weak muscle test means the energy field has been weakened by the offending substance.

But then, how do we use muscle test results in our lives?

Fortunately, what makes the testing indicate different things for different people is also what makes it so very useful. It is up to us to determine exactly what information muscle testing is giving us. Generally the information we get is exactly what we need to know about. To put it simply, let me continue to use my own situation as an example.

When I held a food that would have given me hives, I became totally weak. Did that mean the food was bad for my digestive system? Did it mean I was having an allergic antibody response? Did it mean I would end up challenging my adrenal system by eating it? I still do not know the answers to any of these questions. The extensive medical testing I went through did not pinpoint the problem, and muscle testing simply gave me a yes or no on foods. Eventually an adrenal system problem became the most likely possibility, and I am fairly convinced that is true, but in daily life, that information did not do me much good, since there was no "cure" available. What was useful for my life was just plain knowing that I had better not eat this or that or I would be in trouble. And that is exactly what muscle testing meant for me.

For a long time I hoped muscle testing would help me and the doctors figure out the nature of my problem. I had expected that knowing all the offending foods would give the doctors some clues in treating me. But it turned out that information was not of interest to the allergists at all. It took a while for me to realize the simplest truth, that sometimes it just does not matter exactly *why* there is a problem with a given food or food group. What really matters is to determine exactly what is off limits. And so, at a certain point I stopped analyzing and started simply being amused by the findings.

To get back to the original question, what does the muscle testing really show us? The best answers are in the various stories of people who have gotten weak tests. They seem to fall into several categories.

Allergic types of response:

We already know that muscle testing picks up problems which lead to hives, or other allergic type symptoms like asthma and eczema. Just for background, the "official" allergies, chemically speaking, are immunoglobulin responses, and histaminic body responses. My neighbor, the dermatologist, showed me how during the allergic response state, I had an elevated histamine level that was easy to demonstrate. If I scratched my skin with a fingernail, a red line would appear immediately under the scratch. That was visual proof of my overactive histaminic situation at the time.

Regarding test results, my own story is an example of how a severe case of hives will be predicted by a weak muscle test. My friend, Shelley, whose multiple allergies include asthmatic symptoms, had a breathing problem after dental visits. She tested weak to a latex glove. In her situation, the muscle test was indicating an allergic response to contact in the mouth, without eating or ingesting anything. Another friend had reported that her throat started to close, a more serious but quite common allergic response, during a seafood dinner. She tested very weak to lobster. A weak muscle test could very likely mean a traditional allergy. What else might it mean?

Long term problems:

In the cases of arthritis, in both my mother and my friend Wayne's mother, tomatoes produced a weak test. However, there were no noticeable symptoms after they ate tomatoes. Both women just "loved" tomatoes, and had eaten them frequently in one form or another, fresh or cooked. My mother's arthritis was a much more advanced case, while Wayne's mother's was slight. I cautioned Wayne's mom about eating tomatoes after she tested weak for them and told her about the potential for nightshade vegetables to cause arthritis. She was upset to hear this, and I am honestly not sure whether she has modified her diet because of the test, but at least she has the information to improve and can make decisions knowledgeably.

As for my mother, you may recall from her story earlier that she stopped tomatoes just about completely. But from time to time she would request a test of someone's red sauce at restaurants, hoping her situation had somehow changed. One day she got her result. She started testing strong for tomatoes. In retrospect, it would appear she had a tolerance, a threshold she had exceeded by the quantity of tomatoes she had eaten. Once she stayed off them for long enough, her body became more able to deal with them. At the present time, she will have tomato dishes from time to time and remains strong when tested.

So in these cases, we get two pieces of information. First, that muscle testing can pick up weaknesses which may not have an immediate reaction, but may lead to a long term negative buildup, resulting in ailments like arthritis. Second, that our tolerance can change with time, and with abstinence from allergy-producing foods. In fact, when my own allergies first came out and I spoke to doctors, they explained that an allergic response can be likened to a gas tank, that can hold only so much and then it overfills. Once you go over the edge, the symptoms show up. Then perhaps by eliminating a food for a period of time, the tank empties to such a point that we can go back to having it, but in moderation. What makes muscle testing so wonderful in this situation is that it can be done and done, as often as we wish, and when such a shift takes place, we will know about it and be able to widen our spectrum of foods immediately.

Momentary weakness:

I was once told by a holistic practitioner that muscle testing was not useful because "it keeps changing." From my perspective, however, that is one of its wonderful qualities. It tells you your situation at the moment! In addition to my mother's story above, we have already discussed my friend with irritable bowel, a condition that changes daily. If she used testing on an ongoing basis, she would know which foods were safe at the given time. And there are many of us whose sensitivity level tends to change with the situation.

For another example, most people with allergies tend to become even more allergic while they are in the in the midst of an allergic response. For me there are certain "fringe" foods that I can safely have while I am clear and strong, but if I eat the wrong thing and have a slight case of hives, these questionable foods will become off limits. People whose hay fever is acting up will test weak to more things than when they are clear of the hay fever. Muscle testing tells us our momentary situation, for better or worse. I personally think that is much better.

The role of quantity:

The results of testing definitely reflect the quantity of food being tested. One night my daughter (age 7 at the time) had a big dinner and then decided to eat three oranges for dessert. Her face turned blotchy red. Unsure of the cause, I tested her for oranges — or more specifically, I tested her for an orange. Strong. I tried some of the dinner items. Again strong. Then I got smart and tried two oranges. Still strong. Three oranges? Totally weak.

The story speaks for itself. My daughter now knows not to eat more than two oranges at a time. However, if you have no sensitivity at all to a substance, you will test strong no matter how much of it you have in front of you. There are many instances when we are ever so slightly sensitive to a food and never know about it, because we never eat a large quantity at one meal. Had my daughter decided to have only two oranges that day, I never would have known she had a slight sensitivity to them.

However there is a much more important result to consider. When testing, especially for new medications, for example, holding a whole bottle will test your response for wild megadoses. You want to test for the exact amount you will be taking at the time. Same thing for foods, if you are testing to see if you can have apple cider vinegar and you test weak for the bottle, try again with the amount you really intend to eat.

Location and amount:

Picture this. There I was in the Chinese restaurant, testing a plate of Shrimp and Lobster Sauce. When I was very allergic, the few scallions in the sauce would have caused me to test weak, even though the dish was otherwise okay for me to eat. Knowing that, I would move them to the opposite end of the plate, far enough away to be out of my energy field, we would get the strong test I hoped for and I would safely eat the dish minus the scallions. When I became less allergic, my general strength for the dish overcame the bits of scallion, and I tested strong even with a few pieces of scallion buried in it and close to me. However, if I separated those scallions out and tested a saucer with just the scallions in it, I got a weak result. Very interesting. So what is muscle testing telling us? How can we generalize these results?

First let us discuss location. It is clear that the food within a couple of inches of your "gut" is what is being tested. Regarding quantity, this is a more complex matter. If you are highly sensitive, even a very small amount of an offending substance will overcome anything else in the plate around it (and close to you.) If however, you are basically strong, you might lose some small offending item if it is surrounded by other foods you are strong for. In such a case you might get a strong test result, and still have a small allergic response to the bits of food hidden in the larger dish. To be completely sure, separate out anything you are suspicious of, and test it alone, even in small quantity. But realize that if there is anything in there that is seriously bad for you, it will show up in the testing, even if it has visually disappeared in the sauce.

I would like to finish up with an incident that had us laughing at the time, but has an important lesson in it. I had just come home from a Farmers' Market where I had been with my sister. While there we saw a beautiful display of Texas Onions. These were large white onions with a long green onion top that looked equally delicious. I had bought them because I had amazingly tested strong for them — a true miracle at a time I could not touch even a fried onion, much less a raw one. Still amazed when I got them home, we retested. I held the onions against my stomach by their green tops and basically let them hang. Just then my husband walked in, took one look at me and broke up laughing at the sight of those hanging onions. At the same time my test came out weak. What was happening? After some confusion and several repeats of the weak test, I recalled that I had held the onions sideways at the market. Okay, by then I was willing to try anything. The test with sideways onions was strong. (Can you see why some people think muscle testing is not accurate?) It took a bit more figuring and several repeat tests before the reality became clear — I was allergic to the green tops but not the white bottoms. When I "hung" the onions, it was the green tops that were really in front of my stomach. When I held them sideways, I was really holding the white bottoms against my stomach, and the green tops stuck out to the side, out of the target field. Imagine that!

So the obvious lesson is not about hanging your onions where they don't belong. It is about test location, making sure the exact item you are testing is really in front of your stomach. And, as Felix Unger would say, don't assume. If a vegetable, or anything else has two parts, don't assume all parts are equally safe without a test of each one.

Stomach Intolerance:

This is a condition very commonly indicated by weak muscle testing. For example, my niece mentioned in Chapter 1 had been having powerful stabbing pains every night after dinner. She got negative muscle tests for milk, red meat and tomato products. Once she stopped having these foods, the pains subsided. A colleague of my friend had also been having terrible lower abdominal pains, that often did not let up for days. She tested weak to a large number of seemingly innocuous foods, and when she eliminated them from her diet, started to feel much better after a day or so. To the extent that she really followed through with the restrictions, she remained in less pain. Her case is interesting, because she had some other medical problems which certainly needed to be treated, and I would not suggest that muscle testing eliminated her need for medical treatment. However, it minimized the pain and certainly made her life more pleasant during treatment. Perhaps in her case, the large number of weak foods could have been a clue that a medical problem existed.

For my daughter's six year old friend, the muscle test pinpointed which food was causing a temporary flatulence problem. In her case, there was no pain or noticeable problem other than the smell. However, even that small amount of stomach disruption was picked up by the testing. On the other hand, my own stomach reactions do not appear to trigger weak muscle tests. As I have been becoming less and less allergic, I sometimes test strong for foods that used to cause me hives. Despite the strong test, occasionally I will find myself with an upset stomach right after eating them. In this case, the muscle testing does not indicate the relatively minor weakness, and I am just as glad for that. For me, the upset stomach is a welcome trade off for three days pain of hives, and I am glad muscle testing allows those safer foods not to be confused with the ones that would really make me miserable.

So again the question, what do the results mean? Muscle testing is, indeed, a very individual barometer. We must learn through experience exactly what the test indicates for each of us.

Chapter VIII

What should I test?

The answer to this question is not as obvious as it may seem at first. Of course you will test any food or substance you are suspicious of, but it goes much farther than that. To be aware of all the possibilities for usefulness of muscle testing, you have to have lived with it for some time. In this chapter, I will share with you the benefits of my experience, with my own and other's allergies, and perhaps give you some ideas you would not have had otherwise.

Subgroups and Brands:

When you are dealing with a tool as powerful as muscle testing, you can use it to not only find out what is a problem, but also to maximize your possibilities and find things out you could not have possibly known any other way.

About a year after I started living normally again, thanks to muscle testing, I was in a supermarket buying salad fixings. I knew I could not eat avocados, but this was a store on the Jersey shore that had some fresh produce from farms with large and beautiful stacks of two kinds of avocados. Once again it was my luck that my sister Barbara was with me. She suggested that we give them both a shot. The shiny green ones tested weak. No surprise. I had been off avocados for many months by now anyway. The big surprise was that the nubby black ones tested strong. How nice! I had never considered testing sub-groupings of foods before, but this experience opened up all kinds of new possibilities. I went on to find out that while red apples were off limits to me, green Granny Smiths were okay, although greenish yellow delicious apples were no good. While ripe bananas were no good, under-ripe green ones were okay! I found out that although scallions were no good, leeks were fine.

After being off all hard cheeses for over a year, I learned happily that my favorite, Jarlsburg, would do me no harm. Even my weakness for beef turned up an exception, as I tried testing various cuts and found that flank steak was safe for me to have. As for my husband, he was weak for garlic but somehow shallots were strong. Possibilities opened up before us. Substitutions in cooking became more of a reality.

The next logical thing to do was to test brands, within food types. Some amusing and amazing results came through. We found out that one famous brand name chocolate was the only chocolate I could safely have. Michael, who got migraines after all chocolate, found he was able somehow to have a certain chocolate pudding. (It really does not bother him!) We found that while ham was out of bounds for me, somehow a particular brand named ham was all right. And strangest of all, how could it be that a certain ginger ale was strong for me, while another was weak? I checked the cans and the ingredients were identical. Was this all just whimsy? Was the testing working at all or were we just making this up? No, the weak and strong results remained constant, the same tests produced the same results, even when we could not see the brand names. This was real, and wonderful. How could any doctor, any practitioner, have ever given us this kind of exact information?

The message? Do not assume that just because you have been told you are allergic to apples, berries, chocolate, that you will have problems with all types. Muscle test different types, different brands, different cuts. Get as much variety as possible back into your life.

Hidden foods:

The father of a boy allergic to peanuts told me that his son had to stay away from certain candies because they had peanuts in them. I could not believe it, but it proved true. That was the start of a whole other way of thinking. There are, more often than you might think, foods hidden in other foods. Consider that most Chinese food is fried in peanut oil. Consider that most processed foods are sweetened with corn syrup, or that most light colored sauces are made with chicken stock. Michael (my husband) gets migraines from poultry, yellow corn and peanuts. So far we have found one Chinese restaurant that will accommodate him. The key is that now we know what he needs, and so we can ask for certain ingredients to be included or eliminated.

So the idea is this, if you know you are sensitive to a food that often hides in other foods, test any combination food or any prepared dish that might possibly have something in it that could be a problem. On the other hand, if you are testing a prepared food and it turns out weak, be a detective and try testing its parts individually to see which one is the offender. And look carefully at those lists of ingredients in the supermarket.

Portions:

There are several points here. Firstly, plates of food in restaurants often need to be tested several times, rotating them in order to place different ingredients within the energy field. If a plate of food tests weak, seek further information as to which part is causing the problem. There have been so many times in my own experience when a plate tested weak, but by removing one ingredient, I was able to have everything else on it.

Also, remember that the quantity of food in the field will be reflected in the testing. If you have found a slight weakness by testing one green pea, try testing a full portion before you eat that amount. Do you recall the story of my daughter and the three oranges? Remember what it implies. There are some foods we have slight intolerance for, that we might not ever know about unless we eat an unusual quantity. The best rule of thumb is to test by holding a portion in front of you that is close to the portion you intend to eat.

Being ready for change:

Here is a story that will show you the value of being open mind-ed and ready for change. It involves one of those beautiful platters of vegetable crudites with a dip in the center. Having tested weak for the platter in general, I pushed aside what I knew was a prob-lem, the tomatoes and the blue cheese dip, and started munching. The bartender wanted to know what we were doing, so I picked up the platter to demonstrate a strong baseline. Oh oh! I still tested weak. What now? It was only then that I noticed raddichio being used as a pretty red underlay behind the veggies. Why radicchio is a problem for me I will never know, but I know it is, so off it went, and I tested strong. The bartender was mystified. Now, I could have just nibbled at plain veggies, but I became curious. Maybe the weak initial test had nothing to do with the dip. I sure wanted some. We tested, and found I was no longer allergic to blue cheese dip, at least not this one. Eventually I found I was becoming less and less sen-sitive to most restaurant dips, and by the time of the writing of this book, I am pretty much able to eat most salad dressings. (Of course I still test!)

So, remain open minded, and realize that the answers will not always be what you expect them to be. If in doubt, take the trouble to test, and continue testing from time to time, even items you have been allergic to in the past. Our wonderful bodies do heal, and learn to cope. Things do change!

Medications (including herbal ones):

In the first chapter of this book I told about my mother, who ended up in the hospital with tachycardia after having too much Prednisone. Unfortunately, dangerous side effects seem to be too often the case. It alarms me how often I hear other stories of iatrogenic (physician/medicine-caused) illness, after relating my mother's story.

Here muscle testing is at its most powerful, working literally hand in hand with traditional or alternative medicine to give you the final word on whether to take that capsule in your hand. Its power to give you flexibility is even more crucial in this situation, because it is very often the case that your tolerance to medication changes.

Another instance involving change: After hurting my right shoulder by doing an ill advised stretching exercise, I began taking a few supplements, some calcium, and a pill containing a combination of free amino acids, minerals and herbs, which is supposed to assist in growth and repair of connective tissue. I initially had tested strong for everything and took the combination for several weeks with positive results. Then one day I began to get severe stomach cramps and bowel problems. Immediately, we checked all my supplements and found I was completely weak to the amino acid pill. I stopped taking it for a couple of weeks, having retested weak several times during that period, and of course, felt fine. I say "of course" but imagine what I would have had to do without muscle testing to tell me exactly which pill had caused the problem! I probably would have gone off all the supplements I was taking, including the ones that were helping me and were perfectly in harmony with my system. Then, how to decide whether to go back on any of them?

Eventually one day I tested strong to the amino acid pill, and started to take it again. We continued to test me every day after I took it, and in this simple easy way I was able to let my body tell me exactly what to do.

I am glad to be able to tell the above story using a holistic herbal example. Lest anyone think I am looking to discredit doctors, or allopathic medicine, muscle testing is an individual empowerment tool that is as useful on holistic "medications," as it is on heavy-duty drugs. Although, when using it with herbs, one is more likely to avoid stomach reactions such as mine; with drug-type medications, one is more likely to avoid much more serious and dangerous side effects.

Suffice it to say that before my mother went on blood pressure medication, we tested out the prescribed dosage before she took that first dose. And when it was unavoidable that she take prednisone, we slowly titrated her up in quantity, making sure she was strong all the way. You really need to take it into your own hands. Quite often a well intentioned doctor will say that a dosage is small, but for your body, or your child's or elderly relative's, it might be too much. I have found in my own experience with my mother, that she is extremely sensitive to any medication. Perhaps some older people's systems become more sensitive, more like that of a child. I personally believe that as the baby boom generation enters old age, we will find more attention to exactly that factor. But in the meantime, use your testing to keep your loved ones safe.

One person's cure is another person's poison:

Here is a quick idea for you. I use garlic pills as an antidote for my allergic hives. It was a wonderful discovery, really a gift for me to find something that would stop my hives from developing further, after I had made a mistake. (More on this in Chapter 12) However, we found that my husband is allergic to garlic. In fact, it triggers off migraines for him.

Another quickie - I have been using Echinacea as an early warning cold preventative successfully for some time now. When I saw it sold together with Golden Seal herb, we tested and I found I was allergic to the Golden Seal. Echinacea alone is still fine.

Use this pair of facts as a warning. Just because something is good for one person, don't assume it will be good, or even safe, for another. Test anything new that is to be taken, or anything in megadoses, or anything unusual for the person, even if you think it is great stuff.

Nonfoods:

Although the focus in this book is on food allergies, muscle testing will work perfectly well on substances other than foods. You can use it in the usual way to determine if that type of soap will give you a skin rash, or if a certain lotion or cosmetic will harm you. In one of my supermarket testing sessions, we determined the only safe brand of detergent for a mother to use when washing her allergic son's bedding, by having him hold bottles and boxes of detergent against his stomach.

Once again, the key is for you to remain open minded, and be a detective. Two stories follow, to give you a better understanding:

My good friend Shelley has had severe eczema for many years. When she was a child, she had asthma. Asthma and eczema are two sides of the same allergy — one is on the inside and the other is on the outside. She also has some food allergies. It seems that whenever she visited the dentist, she ended up wheezing. For many years, this phenomenon was basically ignored, as she thought perhaps she was having some fear reaction to dentistry. One day she was reading about latex allergies, and asked me if we could find out with muscle testing whether she was allergic to the rubber gloves. "Let's try," I said, and we took a glove from my husband's office. She tested very weak! We tried washing the powder off the glove, (the staff sometimes complains that the powder irritates their skin) but even the cleaned glove tested weak. When my husband switched to a vinyl glove, her reactions ended. So much for dentophobia! It was a learning experience for him too. Now he checks whether his patients are allergic to latex before assuming he can use regular gloves.

When one thinks about how often latex is used, not only in hospitals and dentist offices, but in more sensitive (ouch!) situations, it becomes a potentially very beneficial thing, to test for latex sensitivity. And yes, it can be done perfectly well by muscle testing.

A more dramatic case: Last winter we were vacationing in Florida with my daughter, whose friend was staying with her grandparents at a lovely condo with a heated pool. It was a cool day, and they had suggested we all come over and enjoy a swim. During a conversation, Michael found out that the grandfather, who was a relatively young and quite powerful man, had been having terrible throat problems and a cough that plagued him. It was not always there, but it kept recurring, and once it began, it would not go away. This had been going on for many, many months. He had been to doctors, and even had an MRI, fearing throat cancer — but no one could find any cause for this persistent problem.

Michael, by now totally indoctrinated in the understanding that muscle testing answers questions, asked the gentleman if he might be allergic to something he eats routinely. Later on, we went back to their apartment to check some suspicious foods in the refrigerator, but everything we tested turned out strong. We were ready to give up, when his wife said quietly, "I wonder if it is my perfume?" He held the bottle, and zingo, his arm dropped with scarcely a push. He protested, saying, "Oh no, this is such nice perfume, I love it!" And he sprayed a puff onto my wrist. Most of it hung in the air between us, and a moment later, as if on cue, he started coughing, sneezing, and his face turned red. He continued to protest, coughing, but one could hardly ignore what was unfolding. She protested too. They really loved that perfume!

I have a funny feeling that she will continue to wear the perfume anyway and he will continue to cough, but at least now they have the information that puts them in control of the situation. And that is exactly what muscle testing does. It gives you knowledge, and puts you in control. What you decide to do after that is your own business!

The fact is that you can test anything that you can hold. If you wanted to, you could test a piece of carpeting by cutting it out and holding it. If something in the carpeting were causing a problem, it would show in the testing. The bottom line again is, keep your mind open and keep testing. After you have adopted a "muscle testing mentality," it will become a way of thinking, a new paradigm, and you will probably end up being able to write your own chapter on what to test.

Chapter IX

Living Happily With the Results

This chapter could also be called, "Now what do I do with this information?" Part of the answer is obvious, you stop having what is bad for you, or at least make an informed decision that it is worth the reaction you may get. However, there is much more to it than that. By now you probably have some ideas on how to live happily with the results, but after having lived it, I can once again make your journey easier by sharing some of the ideas I have picked up along the way.

Coping with Limitations and Realizing Possibilities:

This is actually an extension of what we just said in *Chapter 8* on testing brands and subgroups. Sometimes it is amazing what an allergic person *can* eat. I will never forget my skepticism when I found out that I could not eat tuna, even white tuna, and yet I could eat anchovies, complete with their spicy oil. So I ate anchovy sandwiches for the next three years, or smoked whitefish, which was really a no-pain substitution. Eventually, I found out that a certain brand of tuna was okay, although all the other brands still made me weak. (I will never know exactly when that became a possibility for me, because I never thought to test brands back then.) I used to be a drinker of a certain soda. That became impossible and so I found the joys of another brand. And a funny thing happened. As I became less allergic, I stayed with some of my "new" foods anyway, having gotten so used to them that I enjoyed them better.

I continue to wonder if, even though my body has relearned how to deal with some foods it could not handle in the weaker state, if maybe there is still some stress on my system when I eat foods that once caused trouble. Maybe it is just kinder to stick with things that never bothered me and stay away whenever possible from foods that seem be giving my body some slight stress. It is an open question.

But back to the point, be creative when seeking substitutions — and persistent. One woman had a very strong milk allergy, and so had also given up on margarine, which tends to contain some dairy. When we found a brand of margarine she tested strong for, we noticed thereafter that it had the "U" symbol for "Pareve" on it. This is a verification related to being Kosher, that states the product absolutely has no milk or meat products in it. So, if you are looking for foods safe for lactose intolerance, there is a hint for you. The same woman tested weak to all types of Lactaid (lactose-neutralized milk) except one, the completely nonfat type. So we were even able to find a milk she could have.

Here are a couple of specific suggestions for common allergies. They worked for me and you may want to try them. People allergic to peanuts can often have almond butter instead of peanut butter. Tastes terrific and is a very satisfying substitution. In fact, I have found that people allergic to nuts in general (peanut is not really a nut) often can still have almonds. Another one; when I was allergic to most berries and red grapes, I found that red currant jelly was just as delicious and perfectly safe. Have you realized by now I am leading up to a wonderful substitute for peanut butter and jelly sandwiches? Both my husband and I can eat almond butter and red currant jelly sandwiches. And what a party that first one was!

Of course, I cannot promise that combination will work as well for you. But if not, then use this as inspiration. Just keep trying and you will find there are good things waiting out there to be discovered.

Making Lists:

Life will be easier with a list. You may think you can remember everything, but as you go on, you will find yourself collecting so many little bits of information, brand names, cuts, colors, good substitutions. It really will become a necessity. You will find it invaluable to have that list, if even just for supermarket shopping. So face that fact now and start one at the beginning, before any of your important and quirky information slips away.

Another important use of a list — when you go to a restaurant, you can show it to the waiter. He can use it, even in the kitchen, to check ingredients and give you possible choices for ordering, or to be sure something that will make you miserable has not slipped into the recipe. And so:

Surviving and enjoying restaurants:

Oh, do I have restaurant stories. And each one has a lesson in it. But first the basics:

If you are someone who cares about what the person at the next table may think of you, test while seated, or use the hand method in *Chapter 5* to remain inconspicuous. Of course, by now I hope you will be proud to test publicly, and let the people around you in on this powerful tool. (If you have this book with you, you will appear less flaky to skeptics.)

You may not realize how easy it is to test before you order. Waiters will be happy to bring a spoonful of the sauce, marinade, or gravy for you to check. Be honest and explain you need a bit to see in advance if you are allergic. Reassure them that it is not a problem if the marinade is uncooked or the sauce is cold. And generally it is the unknowns, the sauces, that cause the problem, so you could really clear up some menu possibilities by pre-testing.

If you cannot clear things in advance that way, you can always whip out your list. Choose a dish and a backup, and let the waiter bring your list to the kitchen to see if any forbidden ingredients are present. But remember to test the dish once it comes out anyway. I am sorry to report that even with your best efforts at communication, the accuracy of your directions may not make it to every cook that touches your dish. I cannot tell you how many times a salad has arrived with onions (or worse — the smell of onions, an invisible danger) on it even after we have expressly requested no onions on the salad.

If all else fails, order after someone else gets their dish. This is clearly a last resort, and may not be much fun for main courses, when the whole timing of dinner is affected. But, if necessary, you can get a definite "okay" or a "no" on an entire dish that way, by testing it after it is prepared. And I have gotten around even that inconvenience quite effectively with my husband, who tends to split two dishes with me anyway. If the first dish is okay for us both, we order another and split them both. This way we both get to eat the first half, and at about the right time, the second one comes, nice and hot again.

The "ordering after it is served" alternative is much more useful on desserts, which generally are already prepared and can come right out without delay. You can easily order dessert after some are served, and not feel guilty about making everyone else wait.

Now for the quirky stuff. One night we were at one of those New American restaurants with all the interesting ingredients. You know the ones, black pasta with squid ink in it, ground coriander or its fresh equivalent, cilantro in most of the sauces, spicy Cajun or citrus side dishes — the kind of place Michael and I would have been curious about in our earlier younger lives, but had learned to avoid since developing food sensitivities. But we were there anyway, determined to navigate our way around the menu with lots of testing. It was a small place and we made a lot of friends that night as we tested and people looked.

We were so proud of ourselves as we managed to check the ingredients, discuss options with the waiters who were very forthcoming and get dishes that were not only delicious, but tested strong for us both. Then my nose began to itch....

I panicked. With no idea what I had done wrong, I began to take garlic pills to stop the reaction from progressing further (*Chapter 12* will discuss this more). But since I had no idea what had been the problem, I did not know how many to take. The waiters panicked too. I suppose they did not know what would happen to me next. I explained that it was only hives and I would not explode, but that I really would like to know what had happened.

It was then that our friends spotted the water pitchers at the waiters' station. There were slices of lemon floating in them, a definite "no-no" for me. Can you imagine, needing to test the water? Let this be your warning, if you have any citrus or strawberry allergy. You can never tell what well intentioned restaurant owners will consider to be a special service to customers.

Here is a situation whose lesson is to be sure you know what you are talking about and to test everything. This was a lovely, elegant place. I really trusted the wait staff and really did not want to stand and test. This was also before we had enough practice with seated testing or the hand method to use them discreetly and reliably. So I went over the list, ordered a simple dish with a mushroom cream sauce, omitted the wine and thought I had everything under control. Later that evening the hives hit and I knew someone had done something "wrong." I decided some cook or waiter had poisoned me, and I swore I would never return to that restaurant. It was not until weeks later, when I found I was allergic to mushrooms, that I understood the real truth. I was the one who had "goofed."

At the opposite end of my experiences, there was one local place that saved my sanity. This restaurant would redesign any of their dishes to suit my peculiar list of limitations, and make everything taste great. To this restaurant, and especially the headwaiter, Juan Carlos, who personally oversaw all the wonderful food I had there for close to two years, I would like to express my greatest appreciation. Every highly allergic person like me, who cannot eat most normal foods, should have a Juan Carlos in their life. Once you start dealing with restaurants in these ways, you will have a whole new category in which to evaluate them.

Holiday gift packs from Hell:

This is just to prepare you. If you are one of those people who is allergic to foods, don't get too happy when that pretty mountain of little boxes shows up around the holiday season. It generally contains processed cheeses, nuts, chocolate, strongly cured meats or spicy condiments. I will never forget that year I first became allergic, and after testing over a dozen little boxes and jars, the only thing I could eat was some almonds. I hope you have better results.

And so, if you have a friend who is sensitive to foods, do not send them one of these pretty monsters. It can be depressing. How about a nice fruit basket? No berries or grapefruits please!

Children's happiness:

As any parent of an allergic child knows, it is tricky business to deal with food. There are all kinds of obstacles, from school lunches, to party food, to the inevitable "junk" that becomes the latest food fad. Here are some coping mechanisms to try, after you have fully tested the child and maximized her possibilities.

Send food along. That is the most commonly used solution. It is a way to skirt the issue, and if the child actually sticks with only what has been sent, it works. Unfortunately, it may stigmatize the child, especially if he is the only one with his own bag. Perhaps it would help to tell the child the story of Gloria Swanson, the famous film star of the 1930's, who was way ahead of her time (or perhaps allergic) and brought her health food with her to all the fancy Hollywood parties.

Visit the school and talk to the kitchen staff. You can even come by one day with your child and muscle test the usual foods that are served. At least she will know what is safe to eat, and hopefully have the self-control to limit herself to those foods. Perhaps you can even influence some of the items the kitchen stocks. Similarly for a party, do a little research and find out what will be served. Then go on ahead and pre-test each thing. If the kitchen staff, pizza parlor, or catering facility gives you any trouble about muscle testing, show them this book, to legitimize the validity of what you are doing.

The best way is to empower your child. A child who does muscle testing is a child who will go along with its results. And if your child teaches his friend to test him, well then you have real success. They can test right on the spot. Kids love muscle testing, being naturally open-minded, and they are generally very good at it, having not yet developed a framework of judgments and prejudices. Try giving him/her the power. You might be surprised at how responsible your child becomes about finding his/her own substitutions and controlling his/her own life.

Chapter X

Why do people think this test is
unreliable? - or - It will not work right if...

There are several types of situations in which muscle testing may appear to give inaccurate or unreliable results. In my experience, all of these involve lack of knowledge or understanding by the tester. Any false result can be easily avoided by someone who understands the testing process and is willing to take an extra step here and there to ensure total accuracy. Therefore, this chapter will take an additional step in the direction of troubleshooting the technique, at a more advanced level.

The areas of apparent "unreliability" fall into five categories:

> 1. Neutrality
> 2. Negativity and nervousness
> 3. Strength issues
> 4. Timing
> 5. Accidental sabotage

The following are some incidents which might have led me to doubt the validity of muscle testing. But since I was so personally invested in the procedure, I chose to investigate further instead. The result was that I gained insights, understandings, and improved accuracy.

Neutrality and expectation:

One day, about a year into my odyssey with allergies and muscle testing, I was at a birthday party being attended by my six year old daughter. While talking with the other mothers, I happened to meet the grandmother of the birthday girl. She was an interesting person, a nutritionist with a holistic background. Her daughter had told me that in her earlier years she had done psychic readings, and that she had always been somewhat bohemian in her thinking. Knowing this, I assumed she would be interested in my "life-saving discovery." I explained that I was so thrilled with the results of muscle testing that I intended to write a book about it, to bring this gift to general public awareness.

Her response surprised me. She said she did not hold that much stock in the procedure, because it was unreliable. I responded immediately, and defensively, "It has always been reliable for me!" She said, "But you have to stay neutral." I responded, "I never had to do anything!" I shrugged it off and changed the subject. At that time I was so dependent on my results that I did not want to know about any problems. I simply assumed she was not doing it right, or was just unable to believe it worked. I had encountered the credibility issue often enough with others. So for then, I let it go. But some small lingering question was left in the back of my mind. And circumstance eventually presented another opportunity for me to face the "unreliable" nature of muscle testing.

My sister and mother were at my house, and we were all getting ready to go out to dinner. We were considering what kind of food we wanted. This was the point in time when my mother's tomato weakness had already been determined by muscle testing, but she was asking to be tested regularly to see if perhaps it had gone away. My mother was suggesting Italian food. My sister Barbara, who has done a lot of research into nutritional issues, was dead set against it. She was convinced that the group of foods called nightshades were the cause of Mom's arthritis, and so she just did not want to even test any further. (These foods include tomatoes, potatoes, green peppers, and eggplant.) The fact was, since we had discovered muscle testing, Barbara or I had regularly tested her for various tomato products and she always tested weak. My mother, on the other hand was still hopeful that having been off tomatoes for a long time, maybe she would now be able to have some.

Mom prevailed. So on this evening, we once again took out the can of tomato sauce for testing. I was feeling very open-minded about the issue, after all, it had been a while since my mother had endured an arthritis attack. I tested her for the tomato sauce, and amazingly, she tested strong. Two of the three of us were very happy. My sister was not. She said she wanted to verify my results. Sure, why not? And so she tested my mother for the same tomato sauce, and strangely, she tested weak!

"Of course!" Barbara said, and requested I redo my testing to clarify the issue. I began to doubt the accuracy of my testing. After all, Barbara was the first person who had tested me accurately, and on whose findings I had based my entire diet for many months. How could she be wrong? I must be wrong. Was I pushing hard enough? I tried again, very carefully. I redid the baseline test and found a definite "shelf" where her muscle caught the push. We immediately repeated the motion, with her holding the sauce. I found the same muscle "shelf" holding back the push, a strong test. Was I missing something? I gave her a poke in the left cheek while testing her right arm and the shelf was gone, the arm went right down. No, the test for a weak baseline was definitely giving me a weak result. I retested the sauce. The strong result was clear and definite. At this point I was getting nervous. If two different people were getting two different results, how could I possibly rely on this method, or present it to others? But it *was* reliable for me. That much I knew!

I began to wonder about claims I had heard many years before, from Don, my original muscle tester, that he could predict the result of the muscle test, just before it happened. Lately, my sister was starting to say the same thing, that she seemed to "know" just in advance what the result would be. I have never been particularly psychic, and I am very attached to logic, so I was beginning to wonder whether people who felt they could predict the results were in fact, influencing the results in some way. I suggested this to Mom and Barbara, and they agreed to retest, using brown bags, one with the sauce, another with a definitely safe food. This time around, the results were different, but not totally clear. Barbara's test on tomato sauce was stronger for my mother, although not quite as strong as the safe food. My tests remained the same.

Now it was getting interesting, what could be going on? The words of the holistic nutritionist came back to me, "'You have to be neutral." For sure, my sister had been anything but neutral about the tomato sauce issue, in fact she had become rather upset when my mother originally expressed her preference for Italian food. Pieces were starting to fall into place. We tried another experiment.

I tested my mother again, this time holding nothing. It would ordinarily be a test of baseline muscle strength, but this time, just before I pushed, I thought to myself, "She is going to be weak." Amazingly, she tested weak. Then I did another push. But before doing it, I decided I was just looking for the shelf this time. I said to myself, "Where is that muscle going to lock?" And it did lock, easily resisting the same push that had just brought it down before. My mother now was totally confused, and it was only then that I explained what I had just done.

"Wow, there's something that definitely belongs in the book!" we all agreed.

So, what does this all mean? Do we have to play strange mind games in order to do testing? Does it really show that the method is flawed? This kind of seeming inconsistency is certainly responsible for a number of people who feel muscle testing is unreliable. And yet, when we think about what muscle testing is based on, and use the new paradigm discussed at the start of the book, all this makes sense, and is quite easily manageable.

In short, what weakens the energy field will weaken the test results.

The tester, in assuming something is bad for the person tested, will produce the negative result simply by having that assumption. It would appear that the subtle energy field is negatively affected by this expectation. This fact does create a wrinkle, namely, that a disapproving, dishonest or biased tester can produce false negatives. We must be able to trust our tester.

I thought back to the time I had tested my daughter, then five years old, to a bag of very processed chips and had gotten a weak result. I had strongly wanted her to test weak, and was very pleased when we "proved" the stuff was really junk. Now I would have to go back and redo some of my assumptions. Since then, I have been testing her with a different attitude, and not always getting the answers I would prefer, but I know I am getting the real information. For example, the MSG and chemicals in those chips do not seem to weaken her, and neither does a candy bar. After I got over my disappointment about those facts, I began to realize that maybe I could relax and happily let her enjoy her treats here and there, in the knowledge that they really were not hurting her. And if she does test weak, it is a definite "no-no," something that will likely give her hives or stomach problems.

Okay, so what can we do to make sure we are not having an unintended effect on our test results? Here are a couple of solutions. Try them both and see which is easier for you:

• When you push, think to yourself, "Where is the muscle lock? Let me find that shelf."

• Picture a question mark as you are pushing down.

I prefer to do the first. For me, it is easier to naturally peer off into space as I do a muscle test and just concentrate on the feeling of pressure as I push. Barbara prefers the second. She seems to be more visually oriented. Having a picture of a neutral object that represents questioning is more comfortable for her. Both methods work fine. The idea is to find what you are most comfortable with.

What I find most interesting about this entire issue is that it never was a problem for me in my own allergic situation. The reason I needed muscle testing so badly was also the reason I never had any inaccuracy, namely, we really had no idea what would be good or bad for me. It turns out that in a situation where you really need an answer, when you have no idea what is safe, you will naturally get perfect results with the muscle test. Oh, the beauty of Nature!

Negativity and nervousness:

Let us go a bit further into the idea of testing with paper bags masking the object. It sounds like the solution to the issue of bias, and in fact it can be, if no one becomes nervous in the process. On that day my sister and I were testing my mother, when we put the foods into bags, my sister's testing changed, but still was a bit skewed. She was feeling challenged and starting to wonder if she was going to "get it right." Her results were inconsistent that day, and after a while we all realized that the nervousness engendered by the whole situation was skewing the results.

Earlier in this book I described a situation in which friends mixed up two coffee cups and challenged us to find the decaf. That night I had a moment of alarm, during which I felt pressured to impress them — to "get it right." If I had kept this feeling, it might have confused the results. Perhaps not, but we would have been fortunate to keep a calm energy field in such a challenged state. What happened instead was that we suddenly realized that we no longer knew which coffee was safe for each of us to drink. That became the overriding question, and we easily found our answers because of a real need to find them. That kind of pressure is a pressure to learn the truth, not a pressure of defending our pride or ego. I have always found that when the mind set is "truth-seeking," the results are completely dependable and replicable.

Negativity is another issue. Negativity can ruin muscle testing. Earlier in the book I described the fiasco I encountered when I naively visited my daughter's pediatrician to show him my wonderful discovery. How could I have expected him to accept a procedure that flies in the face of his lifelong paradigm, and just about nullifies at least one area of medical practice? Despite his best intention, he simply could not accept that this could be real. Covert or overt, he had negative feelings about what was happening.

And so, what was the result when I tried to test him? On the baseline, I could not get a clear "shelf." The muscle bounced, and it started to feel like a contest of strength. I should have not even continued, but there was still a lot I did not know at that time. After that, it did not matter what he was holding. With alcohol, poison, I got the same bouncy resistance. At the time I wondered if he was simply too strong. Sensing that this was going nowhere, I covered myself by saying just that, and left with my tail between my legs. For now, let us draw from this the following advice: <u>To test properly, we must start with a clear baseline strength.</u> If we cannot get an easy baseline, we will not be able to make an accurate comparison. And lastly, we must face the fact that there may be some people who simply will not be able to be tested.

Strength and weakness:

It is indeed possible that in the case of my friend the pediatrician, he really had been working out at the gym, and I would not have been able to get a weak response from him no matter what he held. Even then, in a case of extreme strength, when someone is receptive to the testing, I would at least get a definite muscle lock on the strength baseline test first. Someone trying muscle testing and unable to get a weak baseline might conclude the method is unreliable. However, the problem of too much strength can be overcome, as we have already seen in *Chapter 5* under troubleshooting. Here is another example that can serve as a reminder.

One evening I was at a friend's house when her husband's family was over, and I tested weak to her mother-in-law's apple cake. I explained that I could not have it, and she became quite hurt, assuring me that she had used only fresh ingredients and no exotic spices. She was so upset, that I had to elaborate on my entire situation and the test that had just given me the information. This snowballed into a family discussion, as I demonstrated the method to the amazement and entertainment of the whole group. Part of this involved my friend's brother, who clearly was too strong for me to get a weakness baseline.

That situation was easily remedied, using the troubleshooting method given in *Chapter 5*. I stroked against the direction of energy flow, from the ends of the fingers upward on the outside of the arm to the shoulder, a few times. Then I did a baseline for strength (empty hand), and a baseline for weakness (while poking the opposite cheek), both of which now worked perfectly. The upward strokes had temporarily weakened the muscle enough for me to continue testing normally. The interesting part was trying to explain all this hocus pocus to people who had just learned about the muscle test, who were just confronted with the concept of an energy field, and were trying gamely to swallow the whole thing. But they were an open-minded enough group to let it happen. Had I not been so dependent on the method, they might have never been inclined to go so far as to allow or believe in a weakening process. And then they might have also thought the method was unreliable.

One day I was testing my husband, Michael, for a snack he was considering. That day he was involved with a migraine, I believe just getting over one, and he tested very weak for the food. We were suspicious of the result, and so we did a baseline test for muscle strength. There was no muscle lock to speak of, he tested totally weak while holding nothing. In this case, I used the opposite method to strengthen the energy field, stroking in the direction of energy flow from shoulder to the ends of the fingers, on the outside of the arm. After a few strokes, the baseline muscle test produced a nice firm shelf of strength, and the testing revealed he could, in fact, eat the snack.

However, other unexpected things happen, and are probably responsible for a lot of the skepticism among people who are already aware of muscle testing. Take, for example, what happened to me one morning. My sister asked me to test her for some bread. She had already found that bread was weakening her, and had lost weight after eliminating it from her diet. That morning she tested strong for the bread. But we were skeptical of the result. To check it, we tested her for some other breads, ... also strong. Then I grabbed some cleaning fluid. Oh, oh, ... still strong. What now? The solution was straightforward enough, the strokes backward to weaken the energy field. We completed the test, she was still really weak to the bread. But how could this have suddenly happened? Again, if we had not been insistent on making sense of all this, we could have easily abandoned muscle testing as unreliable. After all, why would someone I had tested literally hundreds of times suddenly become so strong?

The answer brings up some interesting questions. It seems Barbara had just come back from jogging and felt wonderful. She has always described the jogging experience as tremendously energizing, yet deeply meditative. The extreme strength of her energy field seems to be testimonial to her description of the experience. In fact, her energy field had become so strong that it had to be mechanically weakened in order to test. In *Chapter 13,* we will take a look at these and other logical conclusions that arise as a result of the recognition of energy fields.

The bottom line of all these experiences? Unreliable results can result from incomplete control of baselines. <u>Always be sure of your baselines, both for strength and for weakness</u>. Re-establish baselines when results seem questionable.

Timing: Getting the "feel" for it and changes in sensitivity:

Some people who have attempted to do muscle testing, give up after a short time and claim that it does not work. In fact, it is just that they have not yet gotten the "feel" and are still unable to do it. It is true that some seem to have a natural knack, and test very accurately with little if any practice. Others have more difficulty. For them it takes a while, but if they continue to attempt testing regularly with a willing (or needy) subject, they eventually catch on. It is very much like riding a bicycle — at some point one gets "a feel" for it, and from then on it comes easily.

In my own experience, my husband, who is an intelligent and capable medical professional, could not test me accurately for weeks. I was completely dependent on my sister during that time. We have discussed possible reasons why he might have not felt comfortable doing this right away, from mistrust, to the possibility that on some level he did not want the responsibility for the decisions made by muscle testing. I would theorize that people who have a great deal of difficulty learning to test have some degree of concern or fear about taking responsibility for what can be some serious decision-making. But that is just a guess on my part. My six year-old also learned to test me with complete accuracy, but again it took some time for the process to jell between us. Perhaps there is really no easy reason. In any case, it is important to keep practicing, and not to give up just because it does not come quickly. Eventually it does come and one has a skill for life.

Timing also comes into play in that some people are stronger or weaker for different things at different times. My friend with irritable bowel syndrome will test strong to green peppers one day and weak the next. Does this mean the testing is unreliable? Some people who are marginally sensitive will have days they are weaker than others. It seems to me that here is the truly magical strength of muscle testing. How else could someone with a fluctuating condition possibly avert problems day-to-day? With traditional allergy testing, a general condition is assessed. Perhaps those people who are tested traditionally will be advised to eliminate a wider than necessary scope of foods to remain comfortable and unafflicted, whereas in muscle testing we find the opportunity to maximize their food possibilities in daily life.

Interestingly, a good friend of my husband's, a professional herbologist and holistic healer, faulted muscle testing for exactly that reason. She said it did not give a dependable result because the results varied at different times with the patient. I understand her point from the perspective of a health practitioner who is attempting to take some overall control of a general situation. However, from the point of view of the afflicted person, who wants to have their own control, muscle testing gives moment-to-moment information that is powerfully valuable.

Accidental Sabotage:

Muscle testing does have some quirks, that can cause false results. (All these have been mentioned in the section on troubleshooting) If you were to accidentally fall into one of the following situations, you might conclude the test does not work.

- Having the tongue pressed against the roof of the mouth, just behind the teeth, will make it impossible to weaken one's energy field. So be sure that the person being tested does not happen to be doing that.

- When testing someone of the opposite sex, do not face each other. Rather, the tester stands behind the person being tested. (If a male faces a female during testing, the male will test stronger than usual and the female will test weaker than usual, which will confound the results.)

And so in conclusion, people who think muscle testing is unreliable are probably people who just do not know enough about the process, or have not given it a full and fair chance. Perhaps they are people who really do not want to know anyway, or people whose belief systems would be too threatened. For those of us who have become knowledgeable enough to make sure our results are accurate, we will know that muscle testing may be "quirky," but when used carefully and knowledgeably gives reliable answers.

Chapter XI

Dealing with Skepticism
and Believing in the Results

In this chapter, we will discuss ways of dealing not only with other people's skepticism, but also with our own. There is a natural tendency, given our common background and upbringing, to discount our findings at some point and even question the validity of the whole muscle testing process. It has happened to me, on and off, at times when my results did not appear to make sense. Other times I just fell back into an old reality paradigm that said, "Could this 'craziness' really be doing something?" But, I have been so dependent on the testing for my physical well-being, and so involved and committed to making it work, that I got past the points of confusion, and inevitably found the problem in testing that produced the strange results. Or I just woke up the next day with my energy paradigm back and said "Of Course this is real."

So know in advance that at some point you may begin to lose trust, for no reason in particular, or know that what may seem to be a wrong result is likely an error in the testing process. Accept the feelings of insecurity, and then try to get past them.

This will likely happen to you even if you do not have a skeptical person around, but the loss of faith will be that much more threatening if you do have someone around you who is not open to muscle testing in the first place, especially one who is offended by the whole thought of a human energy field or "energy medicine." Earlier on we said there are some people who really are just not ready to know about this, and that you and I cannot convert the world. So you may find yourself in the position of having someone you know, perhaps someone close to you, who thinks you are nutty because of muscle testing. If your own confidence becomes shaky and your companion is a strong skeptic, you could lose something valuable.

You have two choices if a significant person in your life is a skeptic: You can let it be, and in your own heart know that you are doing something valid and valuable. In this case, you can send love to the doubter, understand they are not ready and hope they come around one day. Or, one can try to convince or convert the non-believer. The best way to do this would be a demonstration of the strong and weak baselines, if the person's negative energy does not kill off the testing altogether. Then use the explanation of how it works, in *Chapter Six*. If the person is somewhat open minded, you could try simply giving them this book. Somehow when something is out there in writing, it gains more credibility. That is part of the reason I knew this book had to be written. So if you are hesitant about talking to your loved one, try letting the book do it.

It may happen that your break in faith will be caused by something unsettling you may read in the newspaper, or see on an informational television program, such as *20-20* or *NBC Dateline*. In these situations, you need to be armed with the information and logic that will enable you to not be fooled or intimidated. "Logic" can be twisted by "experts," to make a misleading point. Arm yourself against a verbal attack on what you know in your heart and experience is true, by having some logical ammunition ready. Just to set the record straight, I am a mathematician with logic courses in my background, so trust me and follow along. Here is some accurate and comforting logic for you to learn and use, for the benefit of yourself and those you care about.

"Unproven vs. Disproven" - some comforting logic:

There is a common statement that is often used to discredit a method or cure. You have undoubtedly heard it before. Possibly you have heard it from the medical establishment, as a negative response to an alternative technique, herb, or medication. The statement goes like this: "There is no proof that ...(fill in the blank)... is effective in treating the illness. Or the ...(method, herb etc.)... has not been proven effective...," which is logically the same statement. Then the statement might go on to say that the method or herb should be abandoned and those proposing it should not be trusted.

Now, let us look more closely at what is really being said. What this statement actually says is that there is no proof, it has not been proven. But there is no disproof either. Actually, there is no information at all on which to base a decision. The jury is still out — we really do not know anything at all. There is a big difference between *not proven effective* and *proven ineffective*, or between *unproven* and *disproven*. Stop and think about it for a minute. The above statement, and indeed most negative statements about alternative medicine that come from the conservative medical establishment are statements that something is "unproven". (Then the ultra-conservative medical groups tend to begin quacking.) Again, what the statement really means is probably no one has done a double-blind, controlled scientific study at all. Or if studies were done, that they did not meet the "scientific rigor" standards generally discussed in traditional medicine.

We have already looked at the factors working against muscle testing and similar modalities. Who would support such rigorous large scale research? Although things are rapidly and blessedly changing at this time, there are still very few avenues for alternative medicines and techniques to be evaluated in such a way as to be acceptable to the big conservative branch of the medical establishment. And so, yes, muscle testing "has not been shown by research to be an effective method for allergy detection" — at least not in the usual "medical" way. As far as I am concerned, the statement means nothing. Do my successful thousands of tests count as "research?" As "proof?" We have already discussed that question in *Chapter 4*.

So next time you hear some form of that remark, be the smart one, the logician in your group, and explain that "unproven" does not mean "disproven." If something has been subjected to rigorous and "appropriate" scientific scrutiny and has shown itself to be ineffective, that would be "disproven." You see the very big difference.

Invalid studies and reports:

Now get ready for the day you hear there is a study that proves there is no energy field around the body. It is bound to come, and when it does, you ought to know how to deal with it. Why am I saying this? Mostly because of a disturbing series of misinformation I have already seen. In Spring 1998, the prestigious *Journal of the American Medical Association* actually published a "study" designed by a twelve year old girl, (and her conservative-minded nurse mother) that "proved" there was no validity in *Therapeutic Touch*, essentially by "showing" that the so called human energy field could not be detected by a majority of healers when put to the test. Maybe you heard about it. It was very hot news for a week or two.

There are so many holes in that report, which I read carefully, that it became amusing. I won't even bother with all of them. What is most important for us to realize is that the study was designed by a child (?) who had obviously been indoctrinated against energy medicine, who was looking to debunk these healers, and her own hands were used as the "source of energy" to be detected by the therapeutic touch practitioners. Need I say more?

How do I know this? At the bottom of the article, in small letters, it was stated that this study and article was supported by the *National Council Against Health Fraud*, the quackbusting *AMA* subgroup we mentioned earlier in *Chapter 4*, that can only be called reactionary or ultra-conservative.

We know by now that the human energy field is indeed a subtle energy field, and therefore affected by preconceptions, hostility, negativity. I would be amazed if anyone could feel the energy projected by the girl's hand at all. Rather than a situation of an intent to heal, to project love and light, a situation that is present in true *Therapeutic Touch*, this was a contest with a hostile emcee. Her intention to "quackbust" these fakes could easily cause her to project energy erratically, or not at all. The people attempting to test the human energy field knew nothing about how the human energy field functions.

In June 1998, a program on *NBC Dateline* attempted to debunk *Applied Kinesiology*. The reporter and subject were baffled at the sudden weakness of the subject's arm, when her other hand was pointed at certain areas of her body, and so they went to the "expert," to clarify what had happened. And who was that expert? Don't laugh too hard — one of the bigwigs at the *National Council Against Health Fraud*, someone who neither knows nor wants to know anything about the human energy field. Why did they go to a banana expert to ask about oranges? Then the really funny part — he tried to duplicate muscle testing with the subject. Her arm was strong on the baseline, although I saw a lot of bouncing, and he clearly did not have any sense of the feel of the muscle lock. Then he hypothesized that the kinesiologist had hoodwinked her by lifting her arm up higher when he wanted it to weaken. So he tried that, and gee whiz folks, her arm went down. The job was done, *Kinesiology* is a "fraud."

I could not stand it. I started yelling at my family. "He *wants* her arm to go down! He *expects* her arm to go down!" Unfortunately the staff at *Dateline* did not hear me yelling. Even more unfortunately they did not hear my repeated letters, to the Executive Producer, or to a key correspondent involved in consumer and medical issues. But why knock my head against the wall? Is this just another case of people who are not ready? Send them loving thoughts and wait? No. Not this.

The worst part about this kind of "expert research" and reporting is that it can effectively kill off some of the true effectiveness of a therapy or alienate patients who could have previously benefited. For patients whose belief system has been twisted to see energy medicine as quackery, their own negativity, or hostility can adversely affect the energy field around them, if a nurse should attempt the process. Others would not even consent to try. It behooves us all, you too now, to enlighten those around us when news like this shows up.

In fact, the biggest problem with "proving" energy phenomena in traditional scientific ways, is the actual nature of human energy. Traditional scientific research methodology ignores the effects of intention on the results. Double blind is useless if the experimenter is skeptical or hostile to the concept. On the other hand, Quantum Physicists, who are truly on the cutting edge of science, have discovered that very tiny subparticles can respond to the intention of the scientist. When will they all get together?

And there are others, outside the world of conservative medicine, who seem hell bent on discrediting anything having to do with metaphysics in general and the energy field in particular. One of the more visible ones is a magician whom you might have seen in the 50's on television, billed as "Amazing," which his act definitely was. He has, over the last several years, sponsored TV shows that have "dared" psychics and energy practitioners to come on the show and "prove" what they are doing has merit, by offering them large sums of money if they are successful. (Is this in itself a profanation of a previously pure intention? Is anyone trying to demonstrate metaphysics to win big bucks carrying their own negative energy? I honestly do not know.) Invariably they fail and embarrass themselves publicly, and the magician gets the last laugh. Ouch! Once again, there is a highly negatively charged energy situation which has to be getting in the way of any well-intentioned practitioner. It is another hostile emcee, and a powerful one, to boot. Remind me never to demonstrate muscle testing on TV in a "challenge" situation.

Furthermore, he explains that, as a master of illusion, (a good one too!) he is savvy enough to know when phony business is occurring. He then demonstrates what certainly looks like an energy phenomenon, and tells us that it is a carefully designed ruse, a phony. He therefore concludes that anyone doing anything like it is not to be trusted, a charlatan, a quack. Oh, oh! We are back to our logic lesson. His logic in that conclusion is highly flawed. Just because he can create phony energy phenomena does not logically imply that all energy phenomena are phony. I could use the same reasoning to "prove" that all flowers are phony, by producing a convincing silk flower that fools the viewer into thinking it is real. The logic is clearly not there, in the flower situation. Some flowers are fake, some are quite real. It is the same with the energy phenomena the magician demonstrates. Of course fakery is possible, but authenticity is equally possible. Nothing is proven by his demonstrations.

Sometimes I wonder about him. Could he really believe that we are all chumps, being fooled by unscrupulous hucksters? Has his confidence in his own narrow view never been shaken? What would he do if it really were shaken? Print a retraction? He appears to be a well-intentioned private citizen, who for some reason is compelled to save us all. As the King of Siam once said to Anna, "It's a puzzlement."

During one of the news-radio reports on the 12 year old girl's research, I also heard the same gentleman had promised a million dollars to anyone who could "prove" there was a human energy field. When you see him, please tell him that I'd like the money in small bills

So, as you see, there are unfortunately sources at work that for one reason or another, actively fight the expanding knowledge that is coming to so many of us. They are out there, so be aware and be armed with the true realities.

And when you encounter this inevitable report that energy fields are nonsense, or some other such misinformation, be the smart one in your group, the one who understands why such reporting is logically flawed, skewed at best, and perhaps totally invalid. Explain it to your friends, or just pass around a copy of this chapter if you are not in an arguing mood.

People who really do not want to know:

Getting back to the people around you, and types of skepticism you may find as you continue testing, there is a last category of person who may wish to discount your findings. That is someone who simply does not like them. It happened to me on several occasions.

The first was my brother-in-law, who is a very holistic, New Age person, and totally understands about energy, probably more than I do. He was embarking upon a colon cleansing odyssey, with a product that came in several parts for the stages of the program. It was impressively and convincingly written up in the literature that came with the powders, and seemed like a really good idea. But he had begun to have stomach problems. I tested him for two bottles of powder, one was fine but the other definitely weakened him. I suggested he might not have the constitution for this particular program. But he was so "gung ho" on it, he really just could not hear me. What could I do? At that time, and this is a few years ago when my own experience was not as full as it is now, I gave it up. I never asked what had happened, but I recall overhearing he did not finish the program. If this happened now, I would test for portion size, trying smaller and smaller amounts of the powder to try and find an acceptable amount so he could use it. If that did not work, I would still give it up.

Another one, was my friend's father with a known milk allergy. His daughter and wife wanted me to show him why he really should not be having any milk. That was easy enough, his test truly was weak, even when I remained unbiased. "OK, that's nice," he said, "but I am still going to drink the milk, and take my pills." What can one possibly do with that? Could I discuss my philosophy of not putting alien substances into the body or the long term effect of unnecessary drug-taking? The man was close to 80, and robust. Who was I to intrude upon this family argument anyway? I let it go.

Back to my neighbor's tomato-loving mom, first mentioned in *Chapter 7* (on long-term effects, like arthritis.) Ironically, she was the one who wore the perfume that gave her husband the chronic cough, in *Chapter 8*. Well, she did not want to hear about stopping tomatoes, either. Although in this case, I believe she understood what the test was really saying and did cut down, for her own long-term best interest. If I had more continuing contact with her, I would get her to a supermarket to find a type of tomato she could eat without stressing her body.

As one can see, often one will run into people who really do not want to know about the results. But then there are also people who get high cholesterol readings and continue eating fatty foods. These people may be expressing skepticism about the process, or the seriousness of the findings, or may not be skeptics at all, but just do not care about the results.

My advice? If the subject is willing, try to negotiate a middle ground, a smaller portion, a substitution, perhaps. And then let it go and silently send them your best wishes.

Summary:

This chapter has been my most difficult one to write, because it discusses issues that contain so much negativity. Skeptics and skepticism are of many types. Some are caring people around you, with well-intentioned statements of honest disbelief based on lack on knowledge. Or perhaps, they simply come to the situation with their own baggage and needs. Many of those people will be pleased to have a sensible explanation, or if not, they may simply need time. Others are more the power-hungry type, people who might have a "save the world" complex; or whose need to cling to their old power base or belief system causes them to use power in closed-minded and counterproductive ways. Those are the dangerous ones, because they can stand in the way of true progress for us all.

Our role here is to distinguish between the two, and act accordingly. We need to keep our logic and common sense strong, and enlighten people around us when the destructive news stories and "research" results come out. But we do not want to become "fighters" with those around us, who care for us and simply are not ready to understand.

Most of all, we need to relax and let our gut level feelings come through in our own moments of uncertainty, to let us know deep down that this is real, and it is beneficial. And if we know in advance that challenges will come our way, we will be best prepared to handle them.

Chapter XII

Coming Out of an Allergic State

It is an encouraging thought, but what does it mean to "come out of an allergic state?" To naturally grow out of it, or age out of it? To take something to stop an allergic reaction? To cure or end the allergy so it is no longer there? Actually, it means all of those. Let us take a look at them all, and discover how muscle testing will enable you to be in control throughout.

Tracking the process of improvement:

Allergies do not tend to last forever, or even to remain static. We hear about children who grow out of their childhood allergies, and older adults whose allergies end around menopause age. I have been surprised at how often people's allergy stories begin like mine, with some kind of medication that rocks their system. As the body heals, the sensitivities decrease. As for myself, I began to see improvement after about two years, and by the end of the fourth year there were only a few limitations left. Often allergies fade away over time even when they come without a clear cause. As all these changes take place, muscle testing gives us the kind of time-sensitive information one could never get by going to a practitioner. It enables us to maximize our options and live as normally as possible every day.

The idea is simple. As you becomes less sensitive to something, you can track your progress by checking on it any time you like. Just test the portion you would have at the time. As for timing, there are no hard and fast rules about how often to test. The main thing is that you need to be your own detective. If this is a long-standing allergy, you may want to try every month. For a sensitivity that just appeared, like my sensitivity to a food supplement pill, I checked each morning to see if I could take it. Some sensitivities change constantly. My friend with irritable bowel syndrome has a different set of safe foods every day.

What will probably happen naturally is that you will find, from time to time, that a problem food is staring you provocatively in the face, saying, "test me, test me!" And so you will. And some day you will be strong!

Reversing an allergic reaction:

I am not promising this will work for you as well as it does for me, but I have found that a large number of my students with allergies benefit from it. No, I am not talking about any antihistamine which blocks or clouds your body's response. I am talking about the centuries-old natural system cleanser, garlic, and specifically, garlic pills. When you use pills you can easily take a dosage much larger than you could ever eat, without sending your stomach, and your nearby relatives, into shock. My own favorite garlic pill contains 400 mg. of raw garlic concentrate, equivalent to approximately 3750 mg. of organically grown garlic cloves. It is not processed to remove the odor, (processing endangers its effectiveness,) but instead is coated to dissolve only when it has reached the lower intestine, well beyond the mouth and stomach, and so there is no bad odor whatsoever and no bad taste.

Now that you have an idea of the strength of the pill, (check that carefully - there are wide variations) we can discuss how to use it. I have found that garlic pills, taken when I first realize a reaction is beginning, will arrest the progress of that reaction. This means that as far as the reaction has gone, it will go no farther. If I am lucky enough to catch the reaction just as it is starting, garlic pills can even set me back to normal.

But how much to take? There is an interesting question. I will give some general guidelines that work for me, but will they work for you? Here is where muscle testing gives us some amazing information. You can actually use muscle testing to find out exactly how much garlic you need to take to act as an antidote for the amount of offending food you have just eaten.

But first a disclaimer. The antidote test can only be done if you know what you ate that caused the reaction. That can be determined or verified by a muscle test, in which you would hold a similar amount of it, and get the weak result.

The Antidote Test:

While you are holding the same amount of the offending food that caused the reaction, in front of your stomach, have garlic pills in the same hand, also in front of the stomach. When you have reached the number of garlic pills that would counteract the problem, your arm will become strong. Start with one, and work your way up until you find the minimum number of garlic pills that balance out the problem.

The test is so simple, so obvious, and yet so amazingly powerful. I was totally knocked out the first time I thought this up, and it actually worked successfully. And believe me, it does work. I have used it over and over and over, and it really does work. Our bodies have so much information, if only we can figure out how to ask the questions.

Now, what can go wrong? Well, perhaps you do not have an equivalent amount of the food left. Or you are having a reaction to something you had yesterday and you cannot pinpoint just what it is. These conditions make it impossible to test for the correct amount of the antidote, so you will just have to wing it. Fortunately, garlic is really just food, so an overdose will not hurt you. I have found that I have never needed more than four of the above strength pills, and often one or two are enough. After I have taken them, it generally takes no more than 15 or 20 minutes for me to start noticing an improvement in the allergic reaction. In my very worst scenario, I have taken four pills, not knowing for sure, and have ended up with a slight reaction. Even now, if I am somewhere without a tester and I am suspicious of something being served, I will take a garlic pill or two preventatively. That can always be done.

The other problem that can occur with garlic is that some people cannot tolerate it. It is a frustration for me to have this wonderful and easy cure, and not be able to share it with my husband. He tests weak for one garlic pill, and gets migraines from eating raw or even fried garlic. Obviously we cannot use garlic for him, and at this point I have not discovered any other non-medicinal substance that works in quite the same magical way.

Allergy Neutralization - a Cure?

Less than a year after I first discovered muscle testing and left my allergic nightmare behind, I was watching daytime TV and I saw Doris Rapp, M.D., on the Donahue show. She was discussing children's allergies, and how often food can be the culprit responsible for various behavior disorders, including violent behavior problems in children. She showed some graphic footage of a child who was thrashing around, completely out of control,and explained it was the result of a food allergy. This grabbed my attention and I remained glued to the set, as she explained that the sweet child next to her was the same wild one in the film, having been "cured" by a process called *P/N or Provocation/Neutralization*, which had reversed many of his allergies. The mother also explained that during treatment her son had been limited to eating only one food for several months. I wondered if he might have been less painfully limited if they could muscle test him for everything in the supermarket.

Intrigued and sympathetic, with a five year old of my own, I wondered what kind of psychological impact this kind of experience might have for the poor child, even beyond just the physical allergies. I got Dr. Rapp's book, *"Is This Your Child?"* immediately, and read all six hundred or so pages, looking mostly for the description of the procedures that detected and ended the allergies.

Although the major tool for detection was a type of elimination diet,* something that could be easily eliminated itself by the use of muscle testing, the procedure that ended the allergies was fascinating. The provocation/neutralization procedure reminded me of the theory underlying vaccines, that a small amount of an offending substance, when introduced to the body, can in a sense "teach" the body how to deal with it. This rationale also seems similar to that of homeopathy, in which the catch phrase is "like cures like." In P/N, the doctor has to find a perfect small dosage that would not be high enough to cause a reaction. This is generally done by inching upward, using extracts of the food, and injecting them and waiting. The process can take all day, but eventually the ceiling is broken, and the child starts to react, and so the doctor knows the maximum safe dosage was the previous one. This amount is then used to neutralize the allergy, either by injecting it, or by using sublingual drops. The book explains that it takes seven minutes for the neutralization to work.

Highly intrigued, I pondered this situation. The wheels began to turn. Did it really have to take so long? Does a child really have to suffer with needles all day? Can't I do this all without a doctor, in just a few minutes, with muscle testing?

It seemed too simple to believe, but by now I was beginning to understand that a tool like muscle testing routinely makes complicated situations very simple. I tried it that night on myself, feeling

---

*In the basic elimination diet, one begins by eating only one safe food until he/she is clear of allergies. Then one food is added at a time, and very gradually, according to a schedule. In this accurate, but long and tedious way, one can see what food causes a problem. Unfortunately, you may out the hard way, by having to go through a reaction when you find a problem food.

a bit like Dr. Jekyll. We used lemon, a definite allergen for me. I held the lemon and tested weak. I held a small piece and was still weak. I cut the piece in half and was still weak. I cut the half in half again, weak. In half again, weak. Then I became impatient and took one little nib, one droplet of the lemon in my hand. Still weak.

So then I pulled it apart, and kept half of the single nib in my hand, the smaller half. Finally we got a strong test. It seemed there was almost nothing left in my hand, but I carefully put it under my tongue and squished it around there, tasting lemon for the first time in almost a year.

Then we waited. Seven minutes was supposed to be the magic number, according to the doctor. During the seven minutes I had an interesting feeling of almost, but not quite getting a hive. Then it went away. After the seven minutes were up, we wondered, was I cured? Fortunately we had the perfect tool for finding out. So we went for broke. We tested me a whole lemon...and I was strong!

This was just too much. We looked at each other in disbelief. What had we just done? Could I really now eat lemons, or had this process just changed the muscle test? Honestly, I was afraid to eat some and find out. I waited over six hours, retesting periodically to see if I was still strong. I was. Finally I drummed up the nerve to lick a slice, and to even squeeze a bit of juice into my mouth. I waited with garlic nearby. But nothing happened. Nothing.

Well, my friends, that was the last time I was allergic to lemons. I no longer needed any more neutralizations. Also, I found that I was not only neutralized for lemons, but also for orange juice, red apples, grapes and of all things, white wine. Some other less obvious foods came back then too, but I do not recall them accurately enough to put it in writing.

So why do we need the rest of this book? Why don't we all neutralize all our allergies and be done with it? Unfortunately it is not that simple. Depending on the individual, and the food, many protocols are possible, and many levels of response. Dr. Rapp explains that for maintenance, she uses sublingual doses three times a week or one injection once a week. She explains that often the maintenance is needed less and less frequently, and in time could be discontinued. However, sometimes the maintenance protocol remains necessary indefinitely. Often drugs are still needed, but in smaller amounts. (I beg Dr. Rapp's pardon in this very simplified explanation.)

If we translate everything into muscle testing language, what happens is this: Some people are so sensitive to some allergens that it becomes impossible to find a small enough amount as a neutralizer that would give a strong test . Also, neutralizations may work only slightly, or they may only last for a limited time. Fortunately, when you are empowered by muscle testing, you can safely find out to what extent it has worked, whether you are still "neutralized," or if you need another treatment.

In one of my lectures, a gentleman with a severe milk allergy agreed to try a neutralization. He was weak until all the milk was spilled out of the cup, and only the residue was left. We shook it to the edge of the cup, he squished it under his tongue (my official set of directions) and we waited seven minutes. He had become strong for about an ounce of milk. No more. Could he have repeated the process regularly and become increasingly strong? Possibly. How long did it last? I do not know. In that situation, he was not impressed enough with the results to continue pursuing them.

My husband, who cannot eat chicken, decided it was just as well, since he did not care for it anyway. But one night we were at a temple dinner, and his special order fish dish did not show up. Chicken was the only meal left, unless he wanted to have only potato and vegetable. And it smelled really good. He tried a neutralization. We got the safe amount, mashed it flat and mushy, not easy with a tiny amount, and he squished it under his tongue. Seven minutes later he tested strong, and was able to have the entire dinner, no repercussions, no migraine the next day. However, the next time I decided to make chicken, maybe a week later, he was once again weak. It was not a cure, but it did open up the option of trying a neutralization for a one shot meal every so often. He is not motivated enough to try a continuous protocol for more long lasting results. Personally, I wish he would. Maybe when it is time to write the sequel to this book, he will be more agreeable to being the guinea pig.

If we think about it, someone like Dr. Rapp is thwarted in her attempts to help, because she does not have a ready mirror of the situation. Without muscle testing, she would have to guess at which point a patient needs another treatment, and then the patient has to have the appointment to be seen. She has to establish set protocols that work for most people, and then work each person's individual needs into them. Instead you can find your own protocol and determine how successful it has been, all by testing.

Food groups:

When I stopped being allergic to lemon, I also stopped being allergic to several other fruits at the same time. Now I will not pretend to be a nutritionist, and tell you which foods will group together in this way. In fact, my own experience seems to contradict some of the common sense we would make of seemingly similar foods, so I would recommend testing everything no matter what you seem to have become strong for.

To bring this point home, if I had decided I was strong for beef, based on a strong muscle test while I held a flank steak, I could have gotten into a lot of trouble. If you recall, I was somehow able to have flank steak, while still being allergic to most other cuts. Also, the day after I had neutralized for lox (smoked salmon) I was still allergic for a certain brand of tuna, although I remained strong for the lox.

The best and safest way to use the idea of food groups, is for choosing foods to test. If you have become strong for a food, check the others in a group. They might also be strong. Keep testing as time goes by and you are eating the same or similar foods, both to detect slight variations in the category of food, as well as to see if you are still strong.

Staying Safe Throughout:

This chapter has gone farther than the previous ones. We are not only checking the situation and dealing with it, we are attempting to change the situation. It is therefore that much more important that you are in good control of your testing, because you may be deciding to eat small amounts of things you know can hurt you. When I teach a muscle testing class, I do not bring up neutralization the first day. I wait until the class has become confident in their ability to test accurately.

So, let this be a proviso — a warning to anyone trying any of the above techniques. Muscle testing is a wonderful tool, both simple and complex at the same time. There are ways of being sure it is accurate. Do not skip them, use them. Keep going back to the strong and weak baselines, and you will be reassured of accuracy. Understand that you are taking control, and that with control comes responsibility. Enjoy the magic of the process, but do not turn it into a toy or a joke. You and your tester are becoming healers.

Chapter XIII

If Muscle Testing can be real, then what?

Call it an energy consciousness. When you have begun using muscle testing in your daily life, it becomes a part of you. Muscle testing is simple and complete proof of the existence of the human energy field. It shows us in a very concrete way that the energy around each of us is real. The energy field reflects our situation, and can be used to get information. And muscle testing demonstrates that conditions around our body will change the energy field. Will changing the energy field change the body? That is the premise of energy healing modalities like *Reiki* and *Therapeutic Touch*. So many things that did not seem to make sense when we are limited to the old paradigm, now seem perfectly sensible.

Furthermore, through the use of muscle testing, we can see that the quality of energy is real and affected by our emotional state. Shall we prove it right now? Try this with a partner. First get your strong and weak baselines. Now, the subject concentrates on a negatively charged subject. It could be someone very annoying or upsetting, or a very sad or disappointing event. Meanwhile, test the subject and be mentally unbiased. They will test weak.

What you have just demonstrated is that negativity weakens us. If the same person now concentrates on someone they love or a happy event, they will strengthen immediately. We have just demonstrated, in a very black and white method, the power of positive thinking. Imagine that!

I keep reading articles in which patients who have a positive attitude are better able to heal, or recuperate after surgery or a serious illness. Or older people who have animals they love tend to live longer and have decreased disease. So often the doctors or reporters state that while we observe these occurrences, we are not able to explain why or how. But it becomes very obvious, when your understanding of existence includes an "energy consciousness." It makes sense that when we are "down" and surrounded by negative energy we are weaker, and therefore more susceptible to sickness or disease. When we are highly positive, happy or "in love," we are stronger all around. Perhaps we should think twice about what is called the healing power of intention, meditation, prayer and love. It is that same paradigm shift discussed earlier — the shift to an energy consciousness that opens these new horizons, making previously inexplicable things seem possible.

That paradigm shift can cause so many things to look a bit different. In my own life, I find the changes in my thinking to bring me more relaxation and contentment and to cause me to be more and more open-minded. I even see my dog differently. How is it that she knows to bark when a stranger is outside, with all the doors locked and windows closed? How does she know not to bark when I am the one driving up? I highly doubt it has anything to do with smell. It is too far away and the air is too closed off. No. It has to be energy. Watch your dog and learn. When you express real love, and look at the dog with the warmest feelings possible, the tail starts wagging. You do not have to say or do a thing. Love is an energy. My dog knows it without a doubt. Animals seem to have a sixth sense — something we have always heard. Well now we can name it.

Continuing on along the same lines, perhaps primitive man had some of that sixth sense. It would have saved him from getting poisoned in the forest. If we could sense energy we would not need to muscle test. It would be a body awareness, and we would just "know." Perhaps as we have become more complex beings and have pulled away from our direct connections to the land, we have lost most of that sense.

There is a body awareness that some people seem to have more than others. For example, my husband seems to be able to sometimes feel the heaviness in his arm, even before I push on it. He also seems to have an intuitive feel for what foods are not good for him. It is something like a natural aversion to some foods — but a subtle one. When we first got married, I used to make fun of him because he just seemed picky; whereas I was trained to ignore my gut reaction and eat what was supposed to be good. I really thought he was being ridiculously self-indulgent, and that I was doing the "right" thing. Since my allergies, my feelings have come full circle.

After having muscle testing done for about a year, I started remembering how it felt as a child, when I just didn't want to eat something, and I began to notice that many of my allergic foods had an unattractive quality to me. I started to recall my childhood, and my first taste of Coke — not really liking it, but getting used to it because it was supposed to be so tasty. Regarding mushrooms, I recalled my mother would doctor them up with fried onions and a milk gravy — and only then would I eat them. I always thought strawberries were so bitter, but eventually learned to get past that taste. During my allergic period, I could eat none of these. Even now, over four years later, I cannot eat strawberries or neutralize the allergy.

As time goes on, I am paying closer and closer attention to these awarenesses, body awarenesses. And I believe mine are growing. The most tangible example I can give is that I have begun to sense a shift in the way I feel, just before catching a cold. And I sense another kind of shift, when I have been sick and am about to turn the corner and get better. It is almost as if I can feel that corner as it comes. I am glad to be getting back in touch with my body. It feels intuitively to be a good thing.

If we look again at the fact that the negative expectations of the tester cause a negative test result, we get another slant on the power of intention to influence reality. Similarly for the quantum physicists whose particles jump to where they expect them to be. Have you ever read about some super productive businessman who created an empire after starting with very little? There is generally a discussion of his sense of "positive vision," or that he visualized clearly where he was headed while keeping his confident focus on the goal. The success of people like this is well enough documented, although not generally explained logically. When we add the energy field to the equation, the whole idea makes more sense. The positive focus on a clear vision, the concept of visualizing your ideal future, if we consider that these actions might create a kind of energy field that brings that future closer, the idea begins to feel more plausible.

Here is another concept that is related to the new paradigm. Have you ever had the experience that someone you knew was right behind you? It happened to me years ago and I never forgot it. I was sitting in a lunchroom in conversation with someone and I suddenly felt a familiar presence behind me, that I identified with a particular person. Sure enough, I turned suddenly and he was right behind me, about to say hello. In retrospect, I know I felt the energy field. We also have heard about the phenomenon of people who make unmistakable eye contact from opposite ends of a crowded room. Could that be an energy phenomenon?

Where does this all bring us? To a wonderful opening of the minds, and the possibilities, I hope. The fact that you are reading this book says that you have made a decision, to take an active role in your and your family's health and well-being. It is a decision that says, "I can do this." "I don't have to be dependent." And furthermore, "I am open-minded enough to seek information about something that is not commonly part of mainstream knowledge." These are wonderful statements of freedom and independence. You are willing to explore, and you have decided to be in control.

As I have already stated, "with control comes responsibility." If we know that a positive attitude strengthens us, we start to see that there are good reasons to remain as positive as possible. Anger is a trap, it lures us to ventilate that hostility, give some nasty sign to someone on the highway who cuts you off. But if we look at the bigger picture and see that we are weakening ourselves by taking on that negativity, perhaps we will be more likely to laugh it off. Let us teach ourselves and our children that we can influence the atmosphere around us for the better. As we become more and more aware of the power of the mind to create the energies around us, we can actively choose to make that energy more positive every day. We can create a better world, for ourselves, for our family and friends, for everyone.

Tips for Testing Food Groups

If you have no clue as to what foods may be a problem, start testing foods you crave and then try foods which you eat very often.

MEATS AND FISH:
If you test allergic to a type of meat, try different cuts within that group. Also try "dark" versus "light" meats or fish.

VEGETABLES:
Try different colors and types, such as red vs. yellow vs, green peppers and tomatoes. Even a plum tomato may get a different response from a beef tomato — so try all types.
Legumes (peas, beans) may cause allergic response, but all are not the same, do try each type individually.

GRAINS:
Many people are allergic to wheat breads, but pure wheat (shredded wheat type) may be okay.
Corn allergies may not extend to white corn. Also, someone allergic to corn needs to test for anything with corn syrup (in many sweetened foods), or cornstarch (in most Chinese food). If the corn allergy is to yellow corn only, there may not be a problem with the syrup or cornstarch.

FRUITS:
Berries are suspect, but even within that category, blueberries and currants may be okay. Separate.types by colors, the red apples from the green or the yellow.
Green grapes may get a stronger response than red or purple ones. Ripeness may play a factor — sometimes under-ripe fruit are better than fully ripe.

NUTS:
Peanuts are not nuts, but legumes. They can be highly suspect and should be tested.
Some people allergic to most nuts can still eat almonds. Try it.

DAIRY:

This entire category tends to get a thumbs down from many practitioners, however, I have found peoples' tolerance to be widely varied. Try separate categories to see what is okay. For example, there is plain milk, there are sour dairy items (yogurt, cottage and cream cheese, sour cream, etc.), sweet cheeses (mozzarella, ricotta), aged cheeses (hard and soft are separate subgroups which may differ) and ice creams (different brands have different ingredients).

JUNK AND FUN FOODS:

Try different brands, of chocolate or chocolate products, soda, chips, — everything.

About the Author

Elizabeth Spicer is Professor of Mathematics at LaGuardia Community College, City University of New York, where she has taught since 1977. Previously, she taught at Brooklyn College from 1973 to 1976. Her interests include water sports such as snorkeling and sailing, and music, but her greatest involvement, second to Muscle Testing, is in oil painting. Her artwork was exhibited in the 1995, 1996 and 1998 Visual Arts Alliance of Long Island juried exhibitions at Chelsea Center, Muttontown, and on the cover of this book.

Dr. Spicer lives in Roslyn, New York, with her husband Michael, her daughter Melinda, and her dog, Cookie.

For information on Muscle Testing courses, Dr, Spicer may be reached at:

Fax: 516 621-8164
e-mail: Betspicer@juno.com